Atlas

COUNTRY RESOURCES FOR NEUROLOGICAL DISORDERS

2004

Results of a collaborative study of the World Health Organization
and the World Federation of Neurology

Programme for Neurological Diseases and Neuroscience

Department of Mental Health and Substance Abuse

World Health Organization

Geneva

WHO Library Cataloguing-in-Publication Data

Atlas : country resources for neurological disorders 2004.

1.Nervous system diseases 2.Health resources 3.Health manpower 4.Atlases
I.World Health Organization II. World Federation of Neurology.

ISBN 92 4 156283 8   (NLM classification: WL 17)

Printed in France
Designed by Tushita Graphic Vision Sàrl, CH-1226 Thônex

For further details on this project or to submit updated information, please contact:

Dr L. Prilipko
Programme Leader
Neurological Diseases and Neuroscience
Department of Mental Health and Substance Abuse
World Health Organization
Avenue Appia 20, CH-1211 Geneva 27, Switzerland
Tel: +41 22-791 36 21, Fax: +41 22-791 4160, e-mail: prilipkol@who.int

Neurological disorders constitute a large and increasing share of the global burden of disease. Stroke, dementia, epilepsy and Parkinson's disease are important factors determining mortality and morbidity in all societies. However, the resources and services for dealing with these disorders are disproportionately scarce, particularly in developing countries. While neurological service in Western countries varies from 1 to 10 neurologists per 100 000 inhabitants, neurology either does not exist or is only marginally present in major parts of the world.

Over the years, programmes, projects and other activities of the World Health Organization (WHO) in the areas of mental health and neurological disorders have been closely linked. During the past decade WHO has launched a number of global public health projects, including the Global Initiative on Neurology and Public Health, in order to increase professional and public awareness of the global burden of neurological disorders and to emphasize the need for provision of neurological care in first-level and referral health facilities. The outcomes of these endeavours have revealed a paucity of information regarding national and subnational policies, programmes and resources for the treatment and management of neurological disorders.

WHO is responsible for providing technical information and advice to its Member States to help them to improve the health of their citizens. This task is facilitated by collaboration with various scientific and professional groups that have similar goals. The study of country resources for neurological disorders represents a unique collaborative effort between WHO and the World Federation of Neurology (WFN), which is committed to improving human health worldwide by promoting prevention and care of persons with nervous system disorders. WHO and WFN have been working closely for many years on activities related to prevention and control of noncommunicable and communicable neurological diseases. This publication is another product of their close collaboration.

The results obtained from the study of country resources for neurological disorders confirm that the available resources for neurological services in most countries of the world are insufficient compared with the global need for neurological care. The Neurology Atlas presents the facts and figures and highlights the large inequalities across regions and countries, with low-income countries having extremely meagre resources.

The availability of information will lead to greater awareness among policy-makers of the gaps in resources for neurological care. It will assist health planners and policy-makers to identify areas that need urgent attention and to plan the upgrading of resources in those areas. The data also serve as a baseline for monitoring the improvement in availability of resources for neurological care. We hope that personnel involved in caring for people with neurological disorders, including health professionals and nongovernmental organizations, will use the Neurology Atlas data in their advocacy efforts for more and better resources for neurological care.

Dr Benedetto Saraceno
Director
Department of Mental Health and Substance Abuse
World Health Organization

Dr Johan A. Aarli
First Vice-President
World Federation of Neurology

Neurology Atlas © 2004 WHO

◆ The Atlas of Country Resources for Neurological Disorders is a project of WHO headquarters, Geneva, supervised and coordinated by Dr Leonid Prilipko and Dr Shekhar Saxena. Dr Benedetto Saraceno provided vision and guidance to the project. The project was carried out in close collaboration with the World Federation of Neurology (WFN) coordinated by its First Vice-President Dr Johan A. Aarli. Dr Aleksandar Janca provided technical guidance and supervision and was involved in the development of the survey design and questionnaire, data collection and project management. Dr Tarun Dua was responsible for completion of the data collection, data analyses and overall project management beginning 2004. Dr Dua also took the primary responsibility of writing this report. Kathy Fontanilla helped in data management and provided administrative support. Technical and methodological support was kindly provided by Dr Pratap Sharan and Dr Pallab Maulik.

Key collaborators from WHO regional offices include: Dr Custodia Mandlhate and Dr Thérèse Agossou, African Regional Office; Dr Claudio Miranda and Dr Jose Miguel Caldas de Almeida, Regional Office of the Americas; Dr Ahmed Mohit and Dr R. Srinivasa Murthy, Eastern Mediterranean Regional Office; Dr Wolfgang Rutz and Dr Matthijs Muijen, European Regional Office; Dr Vijay Chandra, South-East Asia Regional Office; and Dr Helen Hermann and Dr Xiangdong Wang, Western Pacific Regional Office, all of whom made significant contributions during the development of the project, the identification of focal experts in the area of neurology in Member States, and the review of the results.

The information from various countries, areas and territories was provided by key persons working in the field of neurology identified by WFN, WHO regional offices and the offices of WHO Representatives. The respondents also handled the many requests for clarification arising from the data. The list of the respondents is included at the end of the Atlas.

A number of leading experts in the field of neurology reviewed the project report and provided comments. They include Dr Leontino Battistin, Dr Donna C. Bergen, Mrs Hanneke de Boer, Dr Pedro Chana, Dr Amadou Gallo Diop, Dr M. Gourie-Devi, Dr Jin-Soo Kim, Dr Ashraf Kurdi, Dr Najoua Miladi, Dr Elisabeth Müller, Dr Michael Piradov, Dr Donald Silberberg and Dr Wenzhi Wang. Various specialists contributed short reviews of selected areas in relation to neurology, as follows. Epilepsy: Dr Jerome Engel Jr; Cerebrovascular diseases: Dr B. Piechowski-Jozwiak and Dr J. Bogousslavsky; Headache: Dr Timothy J. Steiner; Parkinson's disease: Dr Bhim S. Singhal; Dementia: Dr Martin Prince; Multiple sclerosis: Dr Jürg Kesselring; Training in neurology: Dr Donna C. Bergen.

A number of colleagues at WHO gave advice and guidance during the course of the project, in particular Dr José Bertolote, Dr Michelle Funk and Dr Vladimir Poznyak.

The contribution of each of the team members and partners, along with input from many other unnamed people, has been vital to the success of this project.

Assistance in preparing the Atlas for publication was received from Tushita Bosonet (graphic design), Steve Ewart (maps) and Barbara Campanini (editing).

There is considerable information available that the global burden of neurological disorders is large and increasing. Very little is known, however, about the resources available within countries to meet this burden. Most information about resources for the care of people with neurological disorders pertains to a few developed countries; little is known at present about the situation in the vast majority of countries, and the information that is available is not comparable across different countries or over time.

To fill this knowledge gap, Project Atlas was launched by WHO in 2000 with the object of collecting, compiling and disseminating relevant information on health-care resources in countries. The first publication of the project provided regional and world figures on mental health resources in an illustrated Atlas of Mental Health Resources in the World 2001. WHO decided to expand the Atlas project into the area of neurology and neurological services, as the next logical step in the work of WHO in assessing country resources – and consequently country needs – to control mental and neurological disorders.

All information and data contained in the Atlas of Country Resources for Neurological Disorders (the Neurology Atlas) were collected from a large international study carried out in 2001–2003, which included 109 countries spanning all six WHO regions and covering over 90% of the world population. The World Federation of Neurology (WFN) collaborated closely in the collection and analysis of the data and the development of the Neurology Atlas, with the active participation of leading experts in neurology all over the world and valuable assistance from WHO regional advisers and WHO country representatives.

The Neurology Atlas illustrates the current status of neurological services and provision of neurological care in various parts of the world. In general, results obtained objectively confirm that the available resources for neurological disorders in most countries of the world are insufficient compared with the known significant burden associated with these disorders. In addition, there are large inequalities across regions and income groups of countries, with low-income countries having extremely scanty resources.

We believe that the information presented in this volume will be useful for a large range of readers including policy-makers, health planners and specialists on international as well as national level. The results of the Neurology Atlas clearly establish the need for substantial increase in the neurology services especially in low and low-middle income countries to decrease the inequity. This would only be possible with significant increase in allocation of financial resources for these services. The data also demonstrate the role of international collaboration and partnerships in making a concerted effort to improve the neurological care.

At the country level, the data summarized in the Neurology Atlas may be used for building up national programmes and development of strategies to improve control of neurological disorders, as well as their implementation at country level. In addition, the Neurology Atlas provides the opportunity for comparative analysis of available resources for neurological disorders across geographical regions and countries.

The material presented is a first snapshot of the actual global situation, and we are aware of gaps in information and possible inaccuracies. We are planning to continue our work in this direction to provide more complete, accurate and comparable information in the coming years.

Dr Leonid Prilipko
Programme Leader
Neurological Diseases and Neuroscience
Department of Mental Health and Substance Abuse
World Health Organization

Dr Shekhar Saxena
Coordinator
Mental Health: Evidence and Research
Department of Mental Health and Substance Abuse
World Health Organization

◆ Very little information exists regarding the country resources available to cope with the known burden of neurological disorders, which is large by all accounts. To fill this knowledge gap, some important information was collected by the headquarters of the World Health Organization (WHO) working in close collaboration with its regional offices and the World Federation of Neurology (WFN). This work was undertaken under WHO's Project Atlas, ongoing since 2000. The Atlas of Country Resources for Neurological Disorders (the Neurology Atlas) describes the global and regional analyses of the country resources for neurological disorders from 106 Member States of WHO, one Associate Member (Puerto Rico), one Special Administrative Region (Hong Kong, China) and one territory (West Bank and Gaza Strip), covering 90.1% of the world population. The information is primarily gathered from key experts in the area of neurology in each country identified by WFN as their official delegates and, in some cases, by WHO regional offices. It is one of the most comprehensive compilations of neurological resources ever attempted. Limitations are to be kept in mind, however, when interpreting the data and their analyses. The key persons were among the most knowledgeable persons in their countries, but the possibility remains of the data being incomplete and in certain areas even inaccurate. The draft report was reviewed by leading experts in the field of neurology and regional advisers of the six WHO regions, and their comments were incorporated. The available literature regarding some of the themes was also reviewed, and the evidence is summarized.

The analyses of the reported frequency of neurological disorders showed that epilepsy, cerebrovascular diseases and headache are among the most common neurological conditions encountered in both specialist and primary care settings globally, as well as in all WHO regions. The other neurological disorders reported frequently include Parkinson's disease, neuroinfections, neuropathies and neurological problems attributable to vertebral disorders. Alzheimer's disease and other dementias were also among the most frequent neurological conditions encountered by neurologists in high-income countries. The programmes dealing with prevention, health care, training of personnel and research in the countries need to be based on locally prevalent disorders.

An important resource is the availability of hospital beds for neurological disorders. Designated neurological beds, though not essential, are an important indicator of the level of organization of neurological services in a country. The median number of neurological beds available in the responding countries is 0.36 per 10 000 population. Two thirds of the responding countries have access to less than one neurological bed per 10 000 population. In terms of population covered, only 8.8% have access to more than one neurological bed per 10 000 population. Neurological beds are particularly deficient in the African and South-East Asia Regions. The median number of neurological beds per 10 000 population in low-income countries (0.03) is much lower than in high-income countries (0.73). Separate neurological hospitals with a large number of beds may not be desirable, but a neurological inpatient facility as a part of general hospital is, however, needed to provide comprehensive neurological management.

Specialized services and personnel are essential to provide comprehensive neurological care. They are also important for providing training, support and supervision to primary health-care providers in neurological care. The median number of neurologists is 0.91 per 100 000 population in the responding countries. This deficiency is particularly evident in the African, South-East Asia, Eastern Mediterranean and Western Pacific Regions. In terms of the population covered, only one quarter has access to more than one neurologist per 100 000 population. The median number of neurologists per 100 000 population is also much lower for low-income countries (0.03) compared with high-income countries (2.96). Recommendations regarding the required number of neurologists in a country are available from countries in the European Region and the Region of the Americas, varying between 1 and 5 per 100 000 population. The number of available neurologists in the low-income countries is very much lower than any of these recommendations.

The availability of other types of highly specialized personnel is also limited, with median numbers for neuropaediatricians and neurosurgeons being 0.10 and 0.56 per 100 000 population, respectively. Again, this deficiency is particularly evident in Africa, South-East Asia, the Eastern Mediterranean and the Western Pacific. In terms of population covered, more than one neuropaediatrician and neurosurgeon per 100 000 population are available for only 2.2% and 15.1% of the population, respectively. Such a situation is particularly evident in low-income countries, with only 0.002 neuropaediatricians and 0.03 neurosurgeons available per 100 000 population.

Neurological nursing does not exist as a specialty in 41% of the responding countries. Three quarters of the responding countries have access to less than one neurological nurse per 100 000 population. The median number of neurological nurses in the responding countries per 100 000 population is 0.11. While training for neurologists is being pursued, specialized neurological nursing training has been neglected even in developed countries.

The presence of subspecialized neurological services indicates the level of organization and development of neurology in a country. Subspecialized neurological services are important, because many neurological disorders require highly specialized skills for appropriate diagnosis and management. Such services also provide the basis for conducting research and training for various neurological disorders. The respondents reported availability of subspecialized neurological services (paediatric neurology, neurological rehabilitation, neuroradiology and stroke units) in at least two thirds of the responding countries for each of these areas. All the subspecialized services are especially deficient in the African Region, while stroke units are also deficient in the Eastern Mediterranean Region. Like all other neurological resources, the availability of subspecialized services is much lower for the low-income countries. In interpreting these data, however, an important limitation should be kept in mind: respondents may have replied positively to the question of availability of subspecialized neurological services in the country even when only a very limited number of such facilities are available in a few large cities, as no information on the type, quality and estimate of number of the facilities was obtained from the respondents.

Basic neurological care, including availability of common drugs, is expected to be available in primary health-care settings. The results show, however, that in 15.6% of the responding countries, not even one antiepileptic drug is available through primary care; the same situation exists in 25% of the low-income countries. Other results show that at least one drug for Parkinson's disease is available through primary care in 60.6% of the responding countries, but 83% of the low-income countries do not have even a single anti-Parkinsonian drug available through primary care. No follow-up treatment or emergency care for neurological disorders is available at primary care level in 24% and 26% of the responding countries, respectively.

Training facilities for neurology are considered an essential part of the health-care system for this specialty in order to continuously improve delivery of neurological care. Although facilities for postgraduate training in neurology exists in 76% of the responding countries, no such facility exists in half of the low-income countries and few are available in Africa and the Eastern Mediterranean. The median number of medical graduates obtaining a specialist degree in neurology every year is 0.04 per 100000 population. The number is much lower in Africa, the Americas, the Eastern Mediterranean and South-East Asia. Although training facilities are available in a large number of countries, the number of postgraduates who obtain a specialist degree is clearly inadequate.

Adequate financing of neurology services is essential to provide the needed care for this group of patients. However, only 10.4% of the responding countries have a separate budget for neurological illnesses within their health budgets. The proportion of the overall health budget allocated for neurological disorders is not specified. Although a separate budget for neurological services is not essential, when present it assists in earmarking the resources and planning the services more effectively. Common methods of financing neurological care include social insurance and tax-based funding (each in one third of the responding countries), followed by out-of-pocket

payments in a quarter of responding countries. Out-of-pocket expenses are particularly important in Africa and South-East Asia. Tax-based funding is the most important source of financing neurological care in the Americas, the Eastern Mediterranean, South-East Asia and the Western Pacific. Social insurance is the most important source of financing in the European Region (58.3% of the responding countries). Private insurance plays very little role in financing neurological care. Out-of-pocket expenditure is the most important method of financing in low-income countries. This is likely to result in more inequity in the utilization of neurological services. Some form of disability benefit is available in 70.5% of the responding countries. However, two thirds of the low-income countries have no disability benefits available. This deficiency is particularly evident in Africa and South-East Asia.

A reporting and information-gathering system for health conditions assists in monitoring the situation over time, alerts the health system to emerging trends, and facilitates planning. A reporting system for neurological disorders does not exist in one quarter of the responding countries and a data collection system does not exist in half of the responding countries. The information collection systems are often not in place in the African, South-East Asia and Western Pacific Regions.

Professional, user and carer groups are among the most influential advocates to improve the quality of health services in a country. Of the responding countries, 87% have a national neurological association; however, only half of the responding countries in the African Region have a national neurological association. These associations are mainly involved in organizing professional meetings and conferences and advising government. Nongovernmental organizations for neurological disorders exist in 71.7% of the responding countries. There are no nongovernmental organizations for neurological disorders in more than half of the responding countries in the Eastern Mediterranean. No such organizations exist in 35% of the low-income countries.

On the whole, the Neurology Atlas data shows that the available resources for neurological disorders in the world are insufficient when set against the known significant burden associated with these disorders. In addition, there are large inequities across regions and income groups of countries, with low-income countries having extremely meagre resources.

Neurology Atlas © 2004 WHO

◆ Fostering cooperation among scientific and professional groups that contribute to the advancement of health is one of the key constitutional responsibilities of the World Health Organization (WHO) (1). In order to fulfil its constitutional obligation, WHO has been collaborating with numerous governmental and nongovernmental organizations and launched a number of international projects that helped health professionals and policy-makers prioritize health needs and design evidence-based health programmes all over the world.

One of the most remarkable collaborative endeavours was the Global Burden of Disease study, which was a result of the coordinated effort of WHO, the World Bank and Harvard School of Public Health. The Global Burden of Disease report drew the attention of the international health community to the fact that the burden of mental and neurological disorders had been seriously underestimated by traditional epidemiological methods that took into account only mortality, not disability rates. This report specifically showed that while mental and neurological disorders are responsible for about 1% of deaths, they account for almost 11% of disease burden worldwide (2).

As the world became aware of the massive burden associated with mental and neurological disorders, it also recognized that the resources and services for these disorders were disproportionately scarce, particularly in developing countries. Furthermore, there has been a large body of evidence showing that, in the years to come, policy-makers and health-care providers in developed and developing countries alike may be unprepared to cope with the predicted rise of the prevalence of mental and neurological disorders and the disability associated with them. In order to respond to this worrisome fact, in 2001 WHO coordinated a large international project aimed at collecting, compiling and disseminating information and data on the existing resources and services for people suffering from mental disorders. This project was carried out by WHO headquarters and involved all six WHO regional offices as well as 191 WHO Member States. The main outcome of the project was the publication of the Atlas: Mental Health Resources in the World (http://www.who.int/mental_health/ evidence/atlas/) that mapped mental health services around the world and provided a snapshot of the situation on the ground regarding this important public health matter (3).

Over the years, WHO programmes, projects and activities in the areas of mental and neurological disorders have been closely linked. Many such disorders are chronic and progressive in nature and fulfil criteria to be recognized as a global public health problem; moreover, they are frequent and disabling, and they represent a significant burden on communities and societies all over the world. The extension of life expectancy and the ageing of the general populations in both developed and developing countries are likely to increase the prevalence of many chronic and progressive physical and mental conditions, including neurological disorders. However, the increasing capacity of modern medicine to prevent death, and the development of new, more effective treatments have changed the frequency and severity of impairment attribut-

able to neurological disorders and raised the issue of restoring or creating life of acceptable quality for people who suffer from their consequences.

In order to increase professional and public awareness of the frequency, severity and costs of neurological disorders and to emphasize the need for provision of neurological care at all levels including primary health care, over the past decade WHO launched a number of global public health projects including the Global Initiative on Neurology and Public Health (4). The outcomes of this large international endeavour, which involved health professionals in numerous countries all over the world, clearly indicated that there was a paucity of information on the prevalence of neurological disorders as well as a lack of policies, programmes and resources for their treatment and management.

In view of these findings and in order to fill the information gap in the area of neurological disorders and services, in 2001 WHO decided to expand the Atlas Project into the area of neurology and to conduct a study of Country Resources for Neurological Disorders. The main objectives of this large international study were to obtain the following expert information:

◆ the most common neurological conditions and their distribution in primary care and specialist settings;

◆ availability of neurological procedures, treatments and services;

◆ number and types of health professionals involved in the delivery of neurological care;

◆ characteristics of postgraduate teaching in neurology;

◆ budget for and financing of neurological care, including the types of health insurance and disability benefits;

◆ availability, role and involvement of national neurological associations and other nongovernmental organizations in advocacy to raise public and professional awareness of neurological disorders and their participation in the treatment, rehabilitation and prevention of neurological disorders.

The study of Country Resources for Neurological Disorders represents a unique collaborative effort, which involved WHO headquarters and regional offices and the World Federation of Neurology (WFN). Although launched under severe staff and budgetary constraints in both WHO and WFN, the project created much enthusiasm and mobilized more than 100 WHO Member States and WFN member societies. The main outcome of the project is the present Atlas of Country Resources for Neurological Disorders (the Neurology Atlas), which provides an illustrative presentation of data and information on the current status of neurological services and neurological care in different parts of the world. It is hoped that the Neurology Atlas will serve as a useful reference guide to both health professionals and policy-makers and assist them in planning, developing and providing better health care and services to people suffering from neurological disorders throughout the world.

All the information and data contained in the Neurology Atlas have been collected in a large international study which was carried out in the period 2001–2003 and included more than 100 countries spanning all WHO regions and continents.

Data collection

The Neurology Atlas is based on the information and data collected by WHO and WFN. At WHO, the work was led by headquarters in close collaboration with the regional offices. The first step in the development of the Neurology Atlas was to identify specific areas where information related to neurological resources and services was lacking. In order to obtain this information, a questionnaire was drafted in English in consultation with a group of WHO and WFN consultants. A glossary of terms used in the questionnaire was also prepared in order to ensure that the questions were understood in the same way by different respondents. Subsequently, the draft questionnaire and glossary were reviewed by selected experts. The questionnaire was piloted in one developed and one developing country and some necessary changes were made. The questionnaire and the glossary were then translated into some of the other official languages of WHO – Arabic, French, Russian and Spanish.

The questionnaire and glossary were sent to the official delegates of all the 90 member societies of WFN. In addition, WHO regional offices were also asked to identify a key person working in the field of neurology in those countries where the WFN liaison person was not available or not responsive. The key persons were requested to complete the questionnaire based on all possible sources of information available to them. All respondents were asked to follow closely the glossary definitions, in order to maintain uniformity and comparability of received information. The Neurology Atlas project team responded to questions and requests for clarification. Repeat requests were sent to the key persons in cases where there was delay in procuring the completed questionnaire. In the case of incomplete or internally inconsistent information, the respondents were contacted to provide further information or clarification; where appropriate, documents were requested to support completed questionnaires.

Received data were entered into an electronic database system using suitable codes and analysed using Stata (special edition) version 8 software. Values for continuous variables were grouped into categories based on distribution. Frequency distributions and measures of central tendency (mean, medians and standard deviations) were calculated as appropriate. Countries were grouped into the six WHO regions (Africa, the Americas, Eastern Mediterranean, Europe, South-East Asia and Western Pacific) and four World Bank income categories according to 2002 gross national income (GNI) per capita according to the World Bank list of economies, July 2003. The GNI groups were as follows: low-income (US$ 735 or less), lower middle-income (US$ 736–2935), upper middle-income (US$ 2936–9075) and high-income (US$ 9076 or more) (5). The countries were also categorized according to the population figures published in The World Health Report 2003 (population data 2002) as: Category I (0–1 million), Category II (1–10 million), Category III (10–100 million) and Category IV (>100 million) (6). The published literature regarding some of the themes was also reviewed and the evidence summarized. The results of the analysis were presented in a draft report which was reviewed by leading experts in the field of neurology and regional advisers of the six WHO regions, and their comments were incorporated.

Representativeness of data collected

Completed questionnaires were received from various WHO Member States, areas and territories: 106 Member States, one Associate Member (Puerto Rico), one Special Administrative Region (Hong Kong, China) and one territory (West Bank and Gaza Strip), which are henceforth referred to as countries for the sake of convenience. The data were collected from 16 countries in the African Region (34.8%), 14 countries in the Region of the Americas (40%), 18 countries in the Eastern Mediterranean Region (85.7%), 43 countries in the European Region (82.7%), 6 countries in the South-East Asia Region (54.5%) and 9 countries in the Western Pacific Region (33.3%). In terms of population covered, the data pertain to 90.1% of the world population; 52.3% of the population in Africa, 89.3% in the Americas, 84.1% in the Eastern Mediterranean, 97.2% in Europe, 96.8% in South-East Asia and 97.1% in the Western Pacific.

Limitations

◆ The most important limitation of the dataset is that only one key person in each country was the source of all information. Although the respondent was a WFN liaison officer and had access to numerous official and unofficial sources of information and was able to consult other neurologists within the country, the received data should still be considered as reasonably and not completely reliable and accurate. In some instances the data are the best estimates by the respondents. In spite of this limitation, the Neurology Atlas is the most comprehensive compilation of neurological resources in the world ever attempted.

◆ Because the sources of information in most countries were the key persons working in the field of neurology, the dataset mainly covers countries where there are neurologists or other experts with an interest in neurology. It is therefore likely that the Neurology Atlas gives an overly positive view of neurological resources in the world.

◆ While attempts have been made to obtain all the required information from all countries, in some countries it was not available. Hence, the denominator for various themes is different and this has been indicated with each theme. The most common reason for missing data was the nonavailability of the information in the country.

- The data regarding reported frequency of neurological disorders in various settings represents an estimate and has not been collected and calculated using stringent epidemiological research methods as for prevalence studies. The data were compared with the published evidence available from various countries and the results of this literature review have been incorporated as separate boxes.

- Certain questions, especially in relation to neurological resources, were framed in such a way that responses could be "yes" or "no". Although this facilitated a rapid gathering of information, it failed to take account of differences in coverage and quality. Respondents may have replied positively to the question of availability of neurological services in the country even if only a very limited number of such facilities were available in a few large cities. Also, the response does not provide information about distribution across rural or urban settings or across different regions within the country.

- It is possible that definitions for various terms vary from country to country. As a result, countries may have had difficulties in interpreting the definitions provided in the glossary. The definitions regarding various human resources, for example, may need to be amended and expanded in future.

- While all possible measures have been taken to compile, code and interpret the information given by countries using uniform definitions and criteria, it is possible that some errors may have occurred during data handling.

Data organization and presentation

The data included in the Neurology Atlas are organized in 15 broad themes. The pages on the right-hand side give a graphic presentation of the data and facing pages on the left provide related text. The graphic displays include maps of the world with colour codings of country data. Regional maps show aggregate figures by WHO regions. Bar and pie charts are provided to illustrate frequencies, medians and means as appropriate. Since the distribution of most of the data is skewed, the median has been used to depict the central tendency of the various variables. Atlas pages also contain definitions of the terms used in the process of collecting the data. Selected findings from analysis of data are described for each of the specific themes. No attempt has been made to provide a description of all the possible findings arising out of data analyses presented. Limitations specific to each theme are to be kept in mind when interpreting the data and their analyses. It should be noted that some implications of the findings for further development of resources for neurological disorders are highlighted.

In addition to the information collected as a part of the Atlas project, the Neurology Atlas also provides some data that were obtained from a review of selected literature under some of the themes. No attempt has been made, however, to provide a comprehensive literature review. This additional information is presented in separate boxes and is shown in a different colour. Brief review of selected topics related to neurology by leading experts is also provided in a separate section.

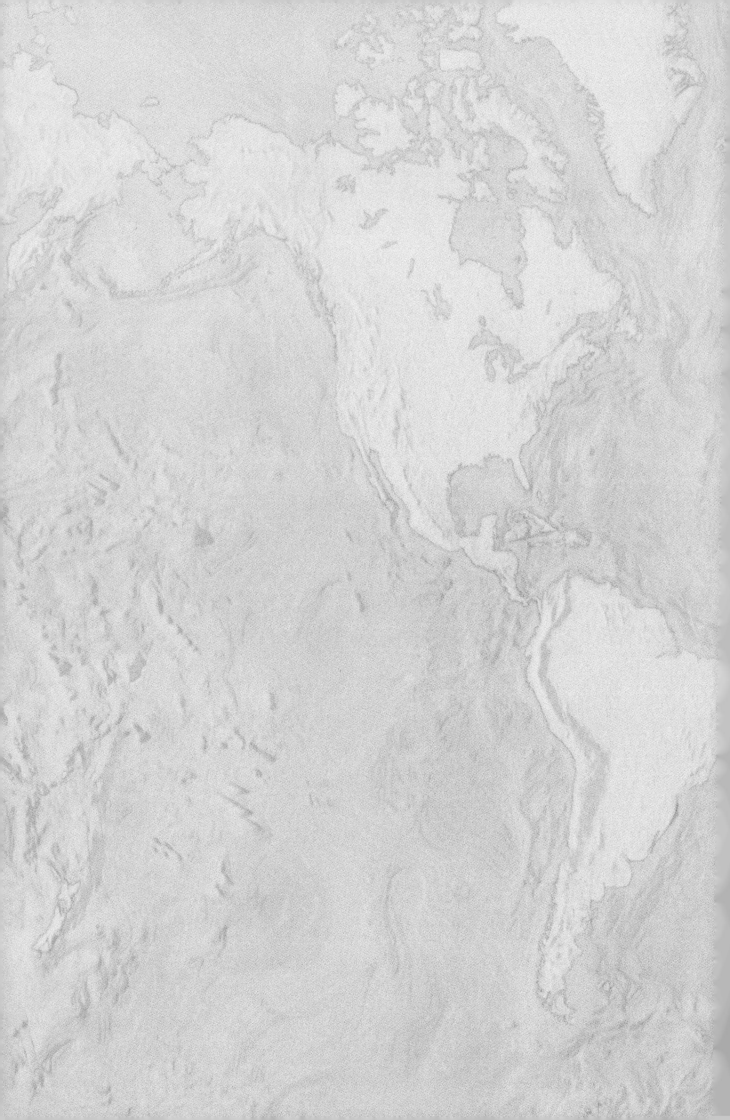

The following pages present
the results of the Neurology
Atlas by themes

REPORTED FREQUENCY

◆ Definitions

◆ **Primary care** in this context refers to the provision of basic preventive and curative health care at the first point of entry into the health-care system. Usually, this means that care is provided by a non-specialist who can refer complex cases to a higher level.

The respondents were asked to provide the five neurological disorders that are most frequently encountered in primary care settings. Ignoring the order of the responses, the proportion of countries that mentioned each of the following diseases was calculated globally and for each of the regions.

◆ Salient findings

◆ Globally, headache (including migraine) is the most common neurological disorder seen in primary care settings (reported by 73.5% of respondents), followed by epilepsy and cerebrovascular disease (72.5% and 62.7% of respondents, respectively). Neuropathies (attributable to diabetes, alcohol, nutritional deficiencies and entrapment) are next in order (45.1% of respondents).

◆ Epilepsy, cerebrovascular disease and headache are also among the five neurological disorders most frequently encountered in primary care settings in all the regions.

◆ Neurological problems caused by vertebral disorders are among the top five neurological conditions encountered in primary care settings as reported by respondents in 34.3% of countries. Neuroinfections (26.5% of respondents), Alzheimer's disease and other dementias (22.6% of respondents) and Parkinson's disease (19.6% of respondents) are the other neurological disorders most frequently encountered in primary care settings.

◆ The top ten neurological conditions seen in primary care settings also included symptoms that had not yet led to a diagnosis such as vertigo, syncope and dizziness (17.6% of respondents).

◆ Limitations

◆ The frequency of neurological disorders in various settings is a rough estimate; data were not collected and calculated using stringent epidemiological research methods as for prevalence studies. The information is based on the experience and impression of a key person in a country and not necessarily on actual data from responding countries.

◆ Although this information is available from only 102 countries, the data represent 90% of the global population. Regionally, the data represent more than 80% of the population for all the regions except Africa, where they represent 52% of the population.

◆ Implications

◆ The information regarding the diseases most frequently seen in primary care settings has implications for making decisions about resource allocation for health care and prevention, research goals, and education of medical undergraduates and general practitioners.

◆ Treatment of common neurological disorders at primary care level would be a cost-effective way of improving the scope and utilization of neurological services.

◆ Integration of neurological care for common illnesses into primary health care is also essential for extending health services to underserved areas in both developed and developing countries.

Review of literature

Headache, epilepsy and neurological problems caused by vertebral disorders featured most frequently (82%, 64% and 64% of studies, respectively) among the top five neurological disorders in the studies describing the prevalence of neurological disorders encountered in primary care settings (7–16). Cerebrovascular disorders and dizziness or vertigo ranked next (36% each). Neuropathies, functional disorders and neuroinfections were also identified among the top five conditions each seen in primary care in 18% of the studies. Parkinson's disease, cranial trauma and psychiatric

disorders (9% each) also featured among the top five neurological disorders seen in primary care settings in some studies.

Cerebrovascular disorders (100% of studies) followed by epilepsy (83%), neuropathies and neuroinfections (67% each) were among the top five admitting diagnoses in the studies concerning the neurological content of general hospital admissions (14, 17–21). The other common reasons for admission included cranial trauma (33%), dementia including Alzheimer's disease (33%), tumours of the central nervous system (17%) and degenerative and demyelinating disorders (17%).

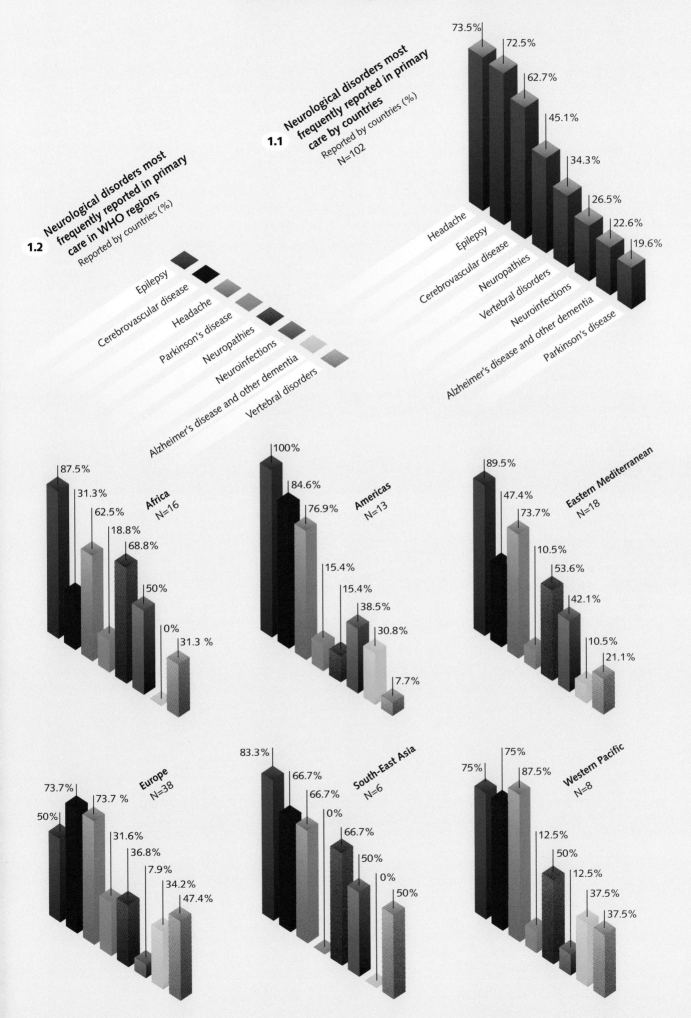

1.1 Neurological disorders most frequently reported in primary care by countries
Reported by countries (%)
N=102

73.5% Headache
72.5% Epilepsy
62.7% Cerebrovascular disease
45.1% Neuropathies
34.3% Vertebral disorders
26.5% Neuroinfections
22.6% Alzheimer's disease and other dementia
19.6% Parkinson's disease

1.2 Neurological disorders most frequently reported in primary care in WHO regions
Reported by countries (%)

Epilepsy
Cerebrovascular disease
Headache
Parkinson's disease
Neuropathies
Neuroinfections
Alzheimer's disease and other dementia
Vertebral disorders

Africa N=16
87.5%
31.3%
62.5%
18.8%
68.8%
50%
0%
31.3 %

Americas N=13
100%
84.6%
76.9%
15.4%
15.4%
38.5%
30.8%
7.7%

Eastern Mediterranean N=18
89.5%
47.4%
73.7%
10.5%
53.6%
42.1%
10.5%
21.1%

Europe N=38
50%
73.7%
73.7 %
31.6%
36.8%
7.9%
34.2%
47.4%

South-East Asia N=6
83.3%
66.7%
66.7%
0%
66.7%
50%
0%
50%

Western Pacific N=8
75%
75%
87.5%
12.5%
50%
12.5%
37.5%
37.5%

◆ Definitions

◆ **Neurological services in primary care** refer to the provision of basic preventive and curative health care for neurological disorders at the first point of entry into the health-care system. The respondents were asked specifically about availability of follow-up treatment and emergency care in primary care settings.

◆ Salient Findings

◆ Follow-up treatment for neurological disorders is available in 76% of the responding countries.

◆ Follow-up treatment facilities for neurological disorders at primary care level are not available in 33.3% of the responding countries in the Western Pacific, 31.2% in Africa, 26.8% in Europe, 23.5% in the Eastern Mediterranean and 7.7% in the Americas.

◆ Emergency care for neurological disorders at primary care level is available in 74% of responding countries.

◆ No emergency care for neurological disorders at primary care level is available in 34.1% of the responding countries in Europe, 25% in Africa, 23.5% in the Eastern Mediterranean, 22.2% in the Western Pacific, 16.7% in South-East Asia, and 7.7% in the Americas.

◆ Limitations

◆ The question specifically requested information about the presence of follow-up treatment and emergency care for neurological disorders in primary care settings. The availability of other basic preventive and curative services was not asked for.

◆ In the event of availability of follow-up treatment facilities and emergency care for even one neurological disorder in primary care settings, it is likely that the question was answered positively. Therefore, the above numbers might be an overestimate regarding neurological services provided in primary care settings. Information on the quality of services and their availability within each country was also not obtained.

◆ The percentage of countries in Europe with follow-up treatment facilities and emergency care at primary care level is low. It is possible that, in many of these countries, the first level of contact as well as follow-up may occur in a specialist rather than a primary care setting.

◆ Implications

◆ Integration of neurological care into primary care is essential in order to extend services to remote and resource-poor areas. The availability of neurological services at primary care level would help in lessening the complications and disability, thus decreasing the burden attributable to neurological disorders.

◆ Many neurological disorders require long-term treatment with drugs and rehabilitation, together with extended and regular health-care contact. Provision of neurological services at primary care level can reduce the burden of these conditions and enhance patients' quality of life.

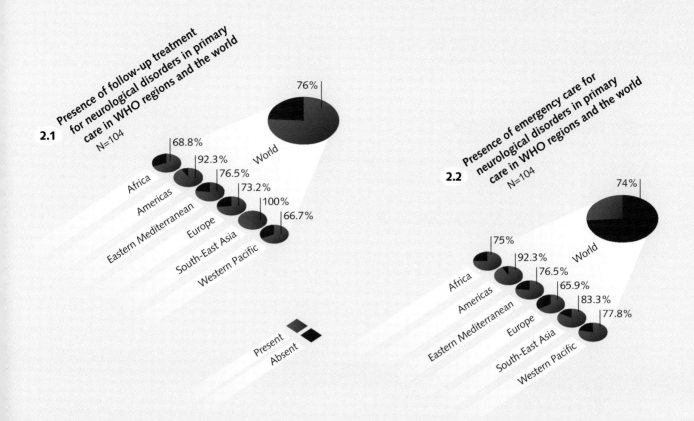

2.1 Presence of follow-up treatment for neurological disorders in primary care in WHO regions and the world
N=104

World 76%

Africa 68.8%
Americas 92.3%
Eastern Mediterranean 76.5%
Europe 73.2%
South-East Asia 100%
Western Pacific 66.7%

Present
Absent

2.2 Presence of emergency care for neurological disorders in primary care in WHO regions and the world
N=104

World 74%

Africa 75%
Americas 92.3%
Eastern Mediterranean 76.5%
Europe 65.9%
South-East Asia 83.3%
Western Pacific 77.8%

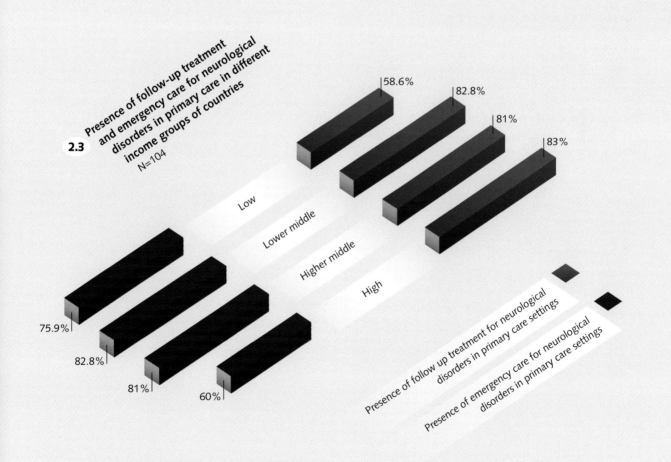

2.3 Presence of follow-up treatment and emergency care for neurological disorders in primary care in different income groups of countries
N=104

Low 58.6%
Lower middle 82.8%
Higher middle 81%
High 83%

Low 75.9%
Lower middle 82.8%
Higher middle 81%
High 60%

Presence of follow up treatment for neurological disorders in primary care settings

Presence of emergency care for neurological disorders in primary care settings

◆ Definitions

- The respondents were asked about the distribution of **essential drugs for neurological disorders** by the government through the primary care system. In countries where the drugs for neurological disorders are reimbursed by the government or social health insurance, they are considered to be available in the primary health-care system.

◆ Salient Findings

- In 22.5% of the responding countries, all standard drugs for neurological disorders are available through the primary health care system.

- Regarding the various groups of drugs, at least one antiepileptic drug (mainly phenobarbitone) is available through the primary health care system in 84.4% of responding countries. In 24.1% of low-income countries, no antiepileptic drugs are available through the primary health-care system.

- Regionally, not even one antiepileptic drug is available through the primary health-care system in 6.2% of responding countries in Africa, 21.4% in the Americas, 10.5% in the Eastern Mediterranean, 18.6% in Europe, 16.7% in South-East Asia, and 22.2% in the Western Pacific.

- Anti-Parkinsonian drugs are unavailable at primary care level in 39.4% of responding countries.

- There is large variation in the availability of anti-Parkinsonian drugs across different income groups: 17.2% of the low-income countries reported the availability of at least one anti-Parkinsonian drug, while 84.4% of the high-income countries reported that at least one anti-Parkinsonian drug is available through the primary health-care system.

- The availability of anti-Parkinsonian drugs through the primary health-care system also varies widely across regions: 12.5% in Africa, 57.1% in the Americas, 73.7% in the Eastern Mediterranean, 79.1% in Europe, 33.3% in South-East Asia, and 44.4% in the Western Pacific.

- Regarding certain other drugs, immunomodulators such as interferons or immunoglobulins for neurological disorders are available through the primary health-care system in 32.1% of the responding countries.

◆ Limitations

- Responses on specific medications were not obtained on a structured format, so there may be some unreliability in the estimates. For example, some drugs (e.g. aspirin) may have been left out.

- Some of the respondents from the European Region reported that no drugs are dispensed by the government through the primary health-care system. This could be a possible reason for the nonavailability of even one antiepileptic drug through the primary health-care system.

- It is also possible that the availability of the drugs is not uniform across primary care centres in a country as information regarding quality of services and availability within each country was not obtained.

- Some of the countries responded that government policy provides for these drugs but financial constraints limit their availability in the primary care setting.

- Availability in a country of even one drug in each category, e.g. phenobarbitone in the antiepileptic drugs, drew an affirmative response. Thus the results fail to differentiate between countries where a wide range of medication is available (e.g. newer antiepileptics) and those where only one or two conventional antiepileptic drugs are available.

◆ Implications

- The nonavailability of drugs in the primary care setting is one of the many reasons for the treatment gap in epilepsy. Because the treatment gap involves much more than the nonavailability of antiepileptic drugs at primary care level, however, other causes – especially related to access and utilization of health services and the problem of stigma – need to be dealt with to decrease the gap.

- The inequity in availability of drugs for neurological disorders across regions and income categories and also within a country needs to be tackled in order to improve the level of primary care for neurological disorders.

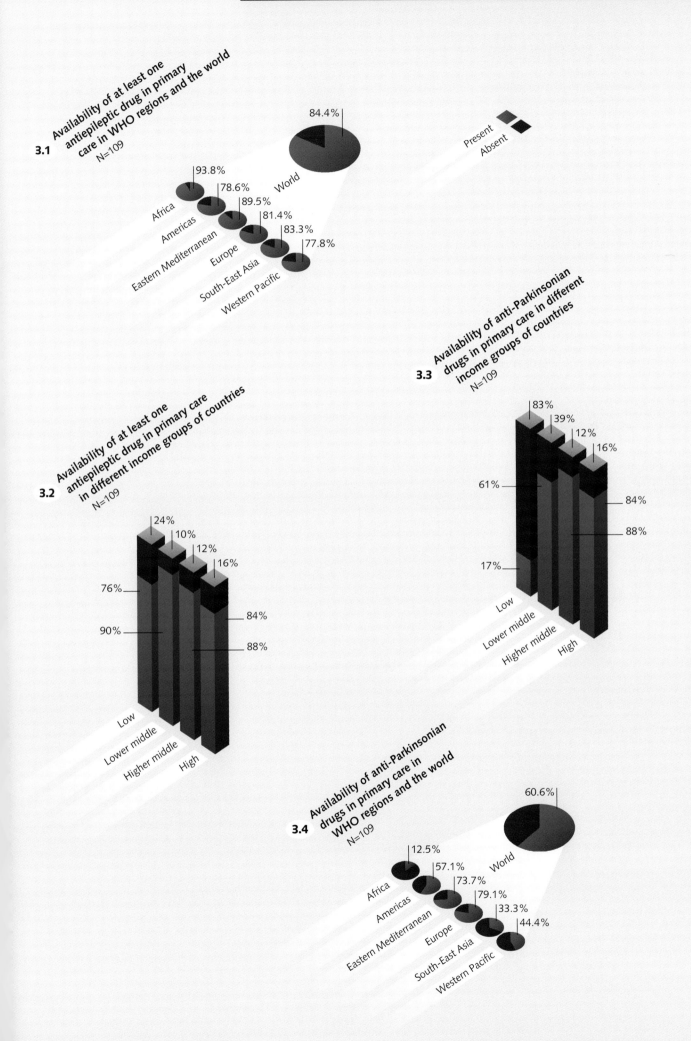

3.1 Availability of at least one antiepileptic drug in primary care in WHO regions and the world
N=109

Present
Absent

84.4% World
93.8% Africa
78.6% Americas
89.5% Eastern Mediterranean
81.4% Europe
83.3% South-East Asia
77.8% Western Pacific

3.2 Availability of at least one antiepileptic drug in primary care in different income groups of countries
N=109

24%
10%
12%
16%
76%
90%
84%
88%
Low
Lower middle
Higher middle
High

3.3 Availability of anti-Parkinsonian drugs in primary care in different income groups of countries
N=109

83%
39%
12%
16%
61%
17%
84%
88%
Low
Lower middle
Higher middle
High

3.4 Availability of anti-Parkinsonian drugs in primary care in WHO regions and the world
N=109

60.6% World
12.5% Africa
57.1% Americas
73.7% Eastern Mediterranean
79.1% Europe
33.3% South-East Asia
44.4% Western Pacific

Definitions

◆ Information on the **neurological disorders encountered by specialists** has implications for health care and teaching. To serve as effective patient advocates, providers of neurological care need to understand the local profile and effects of neurological disorders to plan resource allocation for health care and prevention, neurological care, research goals and medical education.

◆ The respondents provided the five most frequently encountered neurological disorders in specialist settings. Ignoring the order of the responses, the proportion of countries that mentioned each of the following diseases was calculated globally and for each of the regions.

 ## Salient Findings

◆ Globally, epilepsy (92.5%) and cerebrovascular diseases (84%) followed by headache (including migraine) (61.3%) top the list of the diseases most frequently seen by a neurologist.

◆ Parkinson's disease (46.2%) and neuropathies (35.8%) were the other major diseases encountered in specialist settings.

◆ Epilepsy, cerebrovascular disease and headache (including migraine) are also the three top conditions encountered by neurologists in all the regions.

◆ More than one quarter of respondents reported that a neurologist's opinion is sought for Alzheimer's disease and other dementias and in multiple sclerosis.

 ## Limitations

◆ The frequency of neurological disorders in various settings is a rough estimate; data were not collected and calculated using stringent epidemiological research methods as for prevalence studies. The information is based on the impression of a key person in a country and not on actual data from countries.

◆ Although this information is available from only 106 countries, the data represent 90% of the world population. Regionally, the data represent more than 80% of the population for all the regions except Africa, where they represent 52% of the population.

 ## Implications

◆ Major inputs in health care and prevention and priorities for research should be focused on locally prevalent neurological disorders.

◆ The training curriculum of neurologists should concentrate on the prevention and management of these disorders.

Review of literature

Epilepsy, headache and cerebrovascular disorders featured most frequently (88%, 88% and 76%, respectively) among the top five neurological disorders in the studies describing the prevalence of neurological disorders in specialist settings (22–38). Neuropathies and neurological problems caused by vertebral disorders ranked next (36% each). Parkinson's disease and multiple sclerosis were also identified among the top five conditions seen by neurologists in 29% of the studies. Cranial trauma (24%), functional and psychiatric disorders (18% each), dizziness and vertigo, and alcoholism (12% each) and herpes zoster and Down syndrome (6% each)

also featured among the top five neurological disorders seen by specialists in some studies.

Cerebrovascular disorders and stroke appeared among the five most frequent inpatient diagnoses in a study describing the neurological inpatient services in 14 post-communist central and eastern European countries (39). Epilepsy was the second most common diagnosis to feature in the top five conditions in 85.7% of the countries, followed by neuropathies (71.4%), neurological problems caused by vertebral disorders (57.1%) and multiple sclerosis (42.9%).

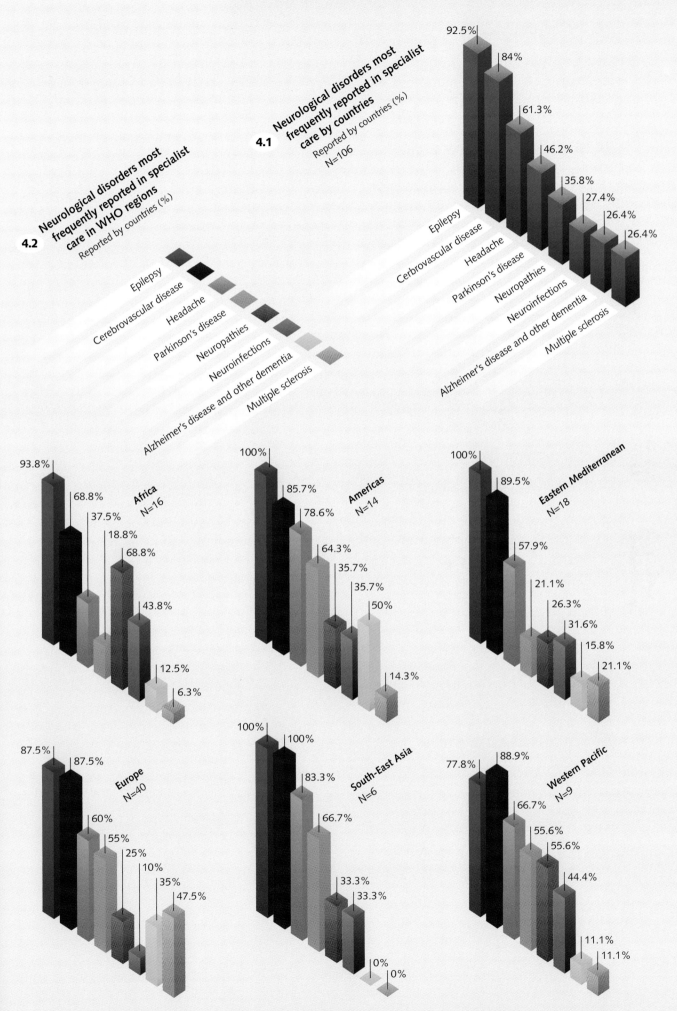

4.1 Neurological disorders most frequently reported in specialist care by countries
Reported by countries (%)
N=106

Epilepsy 92.5%
Cerebrovascular disease 84%
Headache 61.3%
Parkinson's disease 46.2%
Neuropathies 35.8%
Neuroinfections 27.4%
Alzheimer's disease and other dementia 26.4%
Multiple sclerosis 26.4%

4.2 Neurological disorders most frequently reported in specialist care in WHO regions
Reported by countries (%)

Epilepsy
Cerebrovascular disease
Headache
Parkinson's disease
Neuropathies
Neuroinfections
Alzheimer's disease and other dementia
Multiple sclerosis

Africa N=16
93.8%
68.8%
37.5%
18.8%
68.8%
43.8%
12.5%
6.3%

Americas N=14
100%
85.7%
78.6%
64.3%
35.7%
35.7%
50%
14.3%

Eastern Mediterranean N=18
100%
89.5%
57.9%
21.1%
26.3%
31.6%
15.8%
21.1%

Europe N=40
87.5%
87.5%
60%
55%
25%
10%
35%
47.5%

South-East Asia N=6
100%
100%
83.3%
66.7%
33.3%
33.3%
0%
0%

Western Pacific N=9
77.8%
88.9%
66.7%
55.6%
55.6%
44.4%
11.1%
11.1%

◆ Definitions

◆ A **neurological bed** is defined as a hospital bed maintained only for use by patients with neurological disorders on a continuous basis. These beds may be located in public or private neurological hospitals, general hospitals, or special hospitals for elderly people or children.

◆ Salient Findings

◆ A total of 251 455 neurological beds are reported to be available in 95 countries.

◆ The median number of neurological beds in the responding countries is 0.36 per 10 000 population (interquartile range 0.03–1.35).

◆ Almost 70% of the responding countries have access to less than one neurological bed per 10 000 population. In terms of population coverage, only 8.8% of people have access to more than one neurological bed per 10 000 population.

◆ The median number of neurological beds per 10 000 varies widely across regions: 0.03 in Africa and South-East Asia, 0.15 in the Eastern Mediterranean, 0.17 in the Americas, 0.26 in the Western Pacific, and 1.71 in Europe.

◆ The median number of neurological beds per 10 000 population across different income groups of countries also varies: 0.03 and 0.24 for low-income and lower middle-income countries, respectively, while the numbers are 1.83 for higher middle-income countries and 0.73 for high-income countries.

◆ The median number of neurological beds per 10 000 population is higher for countries with smaller populations (0.63 each for countries in population categories I and II) compared with larger populations (0.10 and 0.20 for countries in population categories III and IV, respectively).

◆ Limitations

◆ In many countries, beds are not earmarked for patients with neurological disorders but are part of the pool for internal medicine, neuropsychiatry, geriatrics, paediatrics or general beds; and these may not have been reported.

◆ Moreover, in many countries patients with various categories of neurological disease, e.g. cerebrovascular disease, meningitis, or status epilepticus, are managed on beds allocated to internal medicine, emergency services or intensive care units, and these may not have been reported.

◆ No information is available on beds available in rehabilitation, chronic care or centres for the elderly.

◆ The lower number of neurological beds in high-income countries compared with higher middle-income countries cannot be fully explained. Among the possible reasons are that many high-income countries may not have beds earmarked for the care of patients with neurological diseases, specialized units (stroke units, spinal centres, epilepsy units) are not defined among the neurological beds or there could be other reporting errors. Many of the higher middle-income countries are in central and eastern Europe, where neurological services are well developed and where a broader spectrum of diseases is labelled neurological, e.g. vertebrogenic diseases, and managed in neurological facilities.

◆ Implications

◆ Though not essential for the provision of neurological care, designated beds may be considered to be an indicator of the level of organization of neurological services in a country.

◆ The inequity in neurological services observed across income categories, population categories and geographical areas needs to be specifically dealt with. Separate neurological hospitals with a large number of beds may not be desirable, but a neurological facility as a part of a general hospital is necessary for comprehensive management of neurological disorders.

Review of literature

Very few reports are available (16 countries from the European Region) describing the availability of neurological beds (21, 39, 40). A median number of 3.5 (interquartile range 0.8–7.1) neurological beds per 10 000 population are available in the countries studied. This figure is congruent with the Atlas data wherein a median number of 3.02 (interquartile range 0.4–6.8) neurological beds per 10 000 population are present in these countries. In European countries, recommendations are available regarding the required number of neurological beds: these recommendations vary from 1.5 to 7.3 neurological beds per 10 000 population (21, 41).

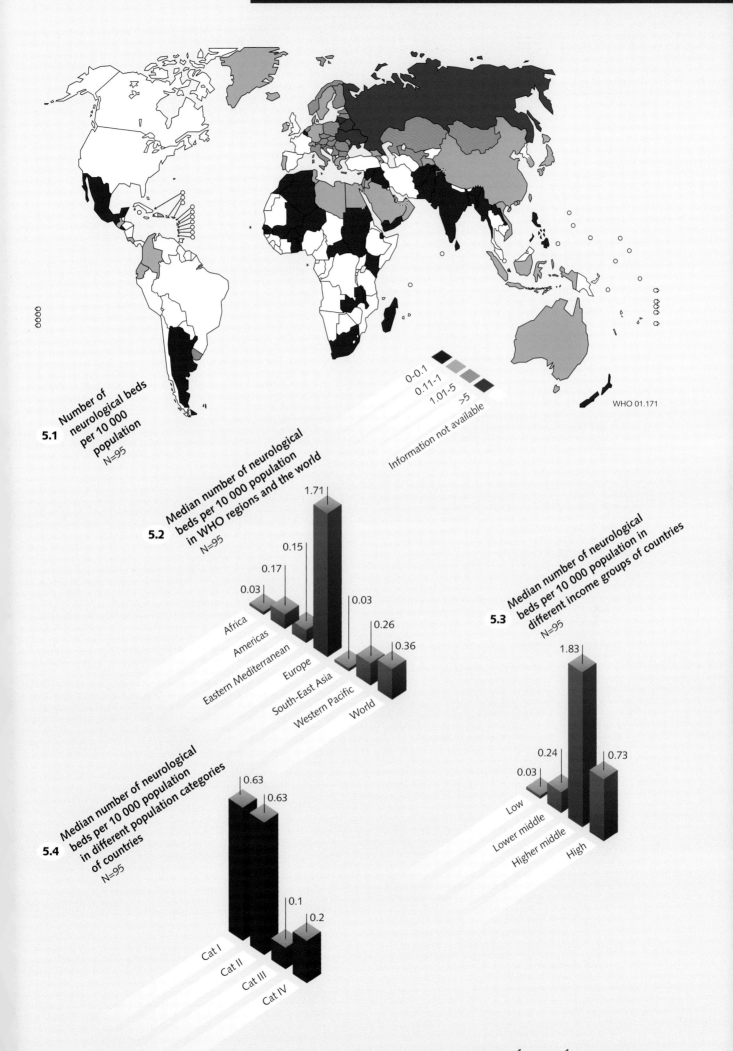

5.1 Number of neurological beds per 10 000 population
N=95

0-0.1
0.11-1
1.01-5
>5
Information not available

WHO 01.171

5.2 Median number of neurological beds per 10 000 population in WHO regions and the world
N=95

- Africa 0.03
- Americas 0.17
- Eastern Mediterranean 0.15
- Europe 1.71
- South-East Asia 0.03
- Western Pacific 0.26
- World 0.36

5.3 Median number of neurological beds per 10 000 population in different income groups of countries
N=95

- Low 0.03
- Lower middle 0.24
- Higher middle 1.83
- High 0.73

5.4 Median number of neurological beds per 10 000 population in different population categories of countries
N=95

- Cat I 0.63
- Cat II 0.63
- Cat III 0.1
- Cat IV 0.2

◆ Definitions

- **Paediatric neurology services** include any hospital, clinic or centre that deals with neurological diseases in children.

- **Neurological rehabilitation services** are team based comprehensive multidisciplinary programmes designed to improve function, reduce symptoms and improve the well-being of patients with neurological problems and their families in their social milieu. These services can be organized as inpatient, outpatient or day-care services.

- **Neuroradiology services** are concerned with the diagnostic radiology of diseases of the nervous system through the use of X-ray, CT scan, magnetic resonance imaging, and angiography and other diagnostic facilities.

- **Stroke units** provide organized care to stroke patients by multidisciplinary teams. They are characterized by coordinated multidisciplinary rehabilitation, staff with a special interest in stroke or rehabilitation, routine involvement of carers in the rehabilitation process, and regular programmes of education and training.

◆ Salient Findings

- Some paediatric neurology service is present in 80.6% of countries that responded. No paediatric neurology services are available in 50% of low-income countries. No paediatric neurology services are available in 62.5% of countries in Africa, 33.3% in South-East Asia, and 31.6% in the Eastern Mediterranean.

- Some neurological rehabilitation service is present in 73.2% of responding countries. In 60.7% of low-income countries, no neurological rehabilitation service is available. No neurological rehabilitation service is present in 81.2% of countries in Africa.

- Some neuroradiology service is present in 77.8% of countries that responded. No neuroradiology services are available in 57.1% of low-income countries. In 81.2% of countries in Africa, no neuroradiology services are present.

- Some kind of stroke unit is present in 62% of responding countries. In 57.1% of low-income countries, stroke units are not available and they are also absent in 25% of high-income countries.

- In 73.7% of countries in the Eastern Mediterranean and in 68.7% of countries in Africa, no stroke units are present and they are also absent in 35.7% of countries in the Americas, 16.7% in Europe, 16.7% in South-East Asia, and 22.2% in the Western Pacific.

◆ Limitations

- Respondents may have replied positively to the question of availability of subspecialized neurological services in the country even if only a very limited number of such facilities are available in a few large cities, as no information was obtained on the type, quality and estimated numbers of such facilities.

- Some respondents may have responded in the affirmative even if the subspecialized services are a part of the general services, e.g. neuroradiology as a part of the general radiological facilities.

◆ Implications

- Subspecialized neurological services are important because many neurological disorders require highly specialized skills for appropriate diagnosis and management. They also provide the basis for carrying out research and training for various neurological disorders.

- The profile of neurological disorders is different in children compared with the general adult population. Special services are, therefore, needed for them as a group.

- A neurological component should be an important part of rehabilitation training of community health workers, because community-based, family-centred and culturally responsive care is the best model to help people with neurological disabilities achieve the highest possible level of function and independence.

- For correct diagnosis and subsequent management of neurological disorders, neuroradiology services are essential. For example, in the case of head trauma, neuroradiology can help to delineate the extent of brain injury or presence of haematoma requiring urgent surgical intervention.

- Substantial evidence shows that organized inpatient care in a stroke unit decreases mortality and residual disability, increases the number of independent survivors and reduces institutionalization, without increasing the cost of care. As these units can be established within the existing medical facilities with minor reorganization of services and training of existing staff without major extra cost to the health-care system, an effort in this direction is required.

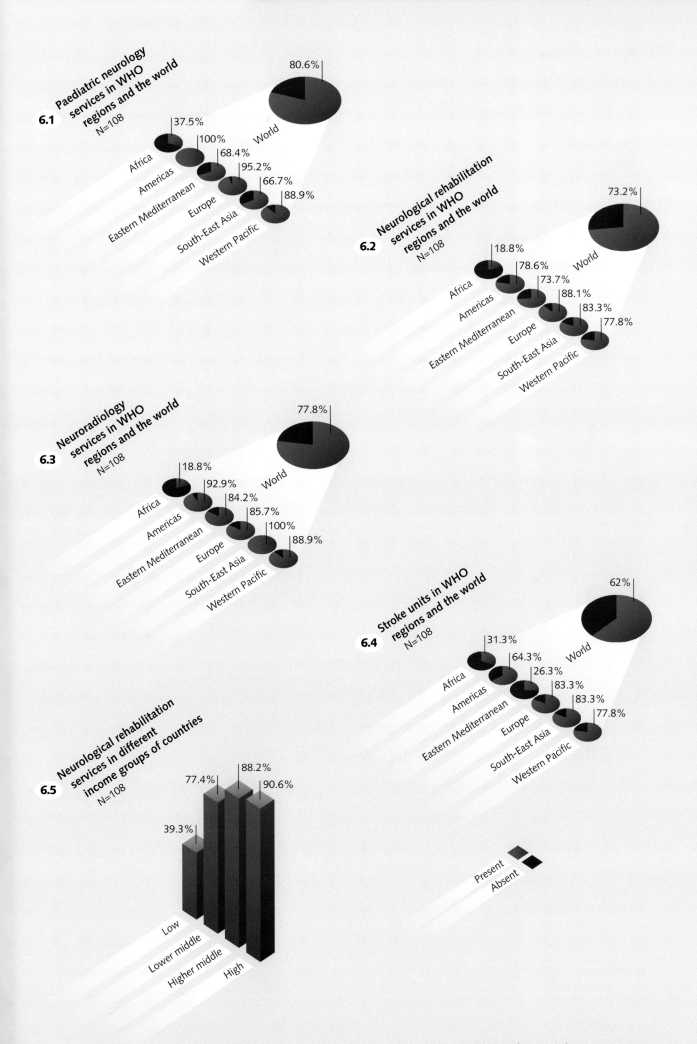

6.1 Paediatric neurology services in WHO regions and the world
N=108

- Africa 37.5%
- Americas 100%
- Eastern Mediterranean 68.4%
- Europe 95.2%
- South-East Asia 66.7%
- Western Pacific 88.9%
- World 80.6%

6.2 Neurological rehabilitation services in WHO regions and the world
N=108

- Africa 18.8%
- Americas 78.6%
- Eastern Mediterranean 73.7%
- Europe 88.1%
- South-East Asia 83.3%
- Western Pacific 77.8%
- World 73.2%

6.3 Neuroradiology services in WHO regions and the world
N=108

- Africa 18.8%
- Americas 92.9%
- Eastern Mediterranean 84.2%
- Europe 85.7%
- South-East Asia 100%
- Western Pacific 88.9%
- World 77.8%

6.4 Stroke units in WHO regions and the world
N=108

- Africa 31.3%
- Americas 64.3%
- Eastern Mediterranean 26.3%
- Europe 83.3%
- South-East Asia 83.3%
- Western Pacific 77.8%
- World 62%

6.5 Neurological rehabilitation services in different income groups of countries
N=108

- Low 39.3%
- Lower middle 77.4%
- Higher middle 88.2%
- High 90.6%

Present
Absent

◆ Definitions

◆ In this context, a **neurologist** is a medical graduate who has successfully completed at least two years of postgraduate training in neurology from a recognized teaching institution.

◆ Salient Findings

◆ In total, 85 318 neurologists are reported to be available in 106 countries. The median number of neurologists in the responding countries is 0.91 per 100 000 population (interquartile range 0.18–4.48).

◆ The median number of neurologists per 100 000 population also varies widely across regions: 0.03 in Africa, 0.07 in South-East Asia, 0.32 in the Eastern Mediterranean, 0.77 in the Western Pacific, 0.89 in the Americas, and 4.84 in Europe.

◆ All responding countries in Africa and South-East Asia, 89% in the Eastern Mediterranean, 67% in the Western Pacific, 50% in the Americas and 7% in Europe have less than one neurologist per 100 000 population.

◆ In terms of the population covered, 25% have access to more than one neurologist per 100 000 population.

◆ The median number of neurologist per 100 000 population across different income groups of countries also varies: 0.03 for low-income countries compared with 2.96 for high-income countries. Even among high-income countries, 24% have access to less than one neurologist per 100 000 population.

◆ The median number of neurologists per 100 000 population is 2.30 for countries in population category I compared to 0.62 in population category IV.

◆ Limitations

◆ Because the sources of information in most countries were key persons working in neurology, the data pertain mainly to countries where there are neurologists or persons with an interest in neurology. It is therefore possible that the above figures might be overestimated.

◆ In some countries, neurological diseases such as epilepsy and dementia are also managed by psychiatrists.

The information from these countries might therefore be an underestimate.

◆ Information about the distribution of neurologists within countries is not available but, as reported by some respondents, the majority are likely to be concentrated in urban areas, thus leading to more inequity than is apparent from the above figures.

◆ Implications

◆ Neurologists are essential in order to provide comprehensive neurological care. They are also important for providing training, support and supervision to nurses, other paramedical staff and primary health-care providers in neurological care.

◆ The inequity in the number of neurologists observed across countries in different income groups, population categories and geographical areas needs to be specifically dealt with.

◆ The appropriate number of neurologists in the population depends upon the structure of a country's health-care system, the way in which primary care is delivered, the role played by specialists, and the geographical distribution of the population. In high-income countries with large concentrations of urban population, the specialists primarily act as clinical caregivers; in low-income countries with large, widely distributed rural populations the most appropriate role for smaller numbers of specialists may be in training and education of primary health-care personnel, and in advising on health care planning.

Review of literature

Reports are available from 67 countries regarding the number of neurologists (32, 36, 42–49). According to the above reports, a median number of 2.5 (interquartile range 0.6–4.7) neurologists per 100 000 population are available in these countries. The figure is congruent with the Atlas data wherein median number of 2.4 (interquartile range 0.5–5.3) neurologists per 100 000 population are present in these countries. Recommendations regarding the required number of neurologists in a country are available from countries in Europe and the Americas, varying between 1 and 5 per 100 000 population. The number of available neurologists in many of the low-income countries is very much lower than any of these recommendations.

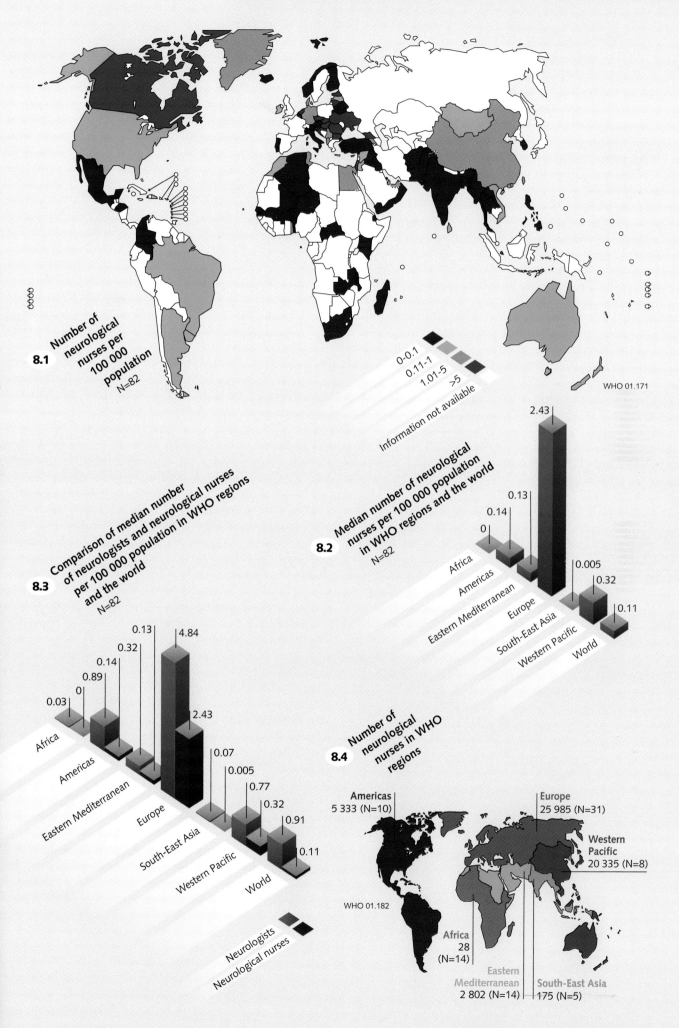

8.1 Number of neurological nurses per 100 000 population
N=82

0-0.1
0.11-1
1.01-5
>5
Information not available

WHO 01.171

8.2 Median number of neurological nurses per 100 000 population in WHO regions and the world
N=82

- Africa: 0
- Americas: 0.14
- Eastern Mediterranean: 0.13
- Europe: 2.43
- South-East Asia: 0.005
- Western Pacific: 0.32
- World: 0.11

8.3 Comparison of median number of neurologists and neurological nurses per 100 000 population in WHO regions and the world
N=82

- Africa: 0.03 / 0
- Americas: 0.89 / 0.14
- Eastern Mediterranean: 0.32 / 0.13
- Europe: 4.84 / 2.43
- South-East Asia: 0.07 / 0.005
- Western Pacific: 0.77 / 0.32
- World: 0.91 / 0.11

Neurologists
Neurological nurses

8.4 Number of neurological nurses in WHO regions

Americas
5 333 (N=10)

Europe
25 985 (N=31)

Western Pacific
20 335 (N=8)

Africa
28
(N=14)

Eastern Mediterranean
2 802 (N=14)

South-East Asia
175 (N=5)

WHO 01.182

◆ Definitions

◆ In this context, a **neurosurgeon** is a medical graduate who has completed at least two years of recognized post-graduate training in neurosurgery.

◆ Salient Findings

◆ A total of 33 193 neurosurgeons are reported to be available in 103 countries. The median number of neurosurgeons in the responding countries is 0.56 per 100 000 population (interquartile range 0.07–1.02).

◆ The distribution of neurosurgeons across regions is variable. The median number of neurosurgeons per 100 000 population is 0.01 in Africa, 0.03 in South-East Asia, 0.37 in the Eastern Mediterranean, 0.39 in the Western Pacific, 0.76 in the Americas, and 1.02 in Europe.

◆ Of the responding countries, 26% have access to more than one neurosurgeon per 100 000 population. In terms of population covered, more than one neurosurgeon per 100 000 population is available for 20.3% of the population.

◆ The median number of neurosurgeons per 100 000 population across different income groups of countries varies. It is 0.03 for low-income countries and 0.97 for high-income countries. Half of the high-income group of responding countries have access to less than one neurosurgeon per 100 000 population.

◆ The median number of neurosurgeons per 100 000 population is 0.94 for countries in population category I, compared with 0.49 for countries in population category IV.

◆ Limitations

◆ Because the source of information in most countries was the professional association, it is possible that neurosurgeons who are not members of these associations were not counted.

◆ Information about the geographical distribution of neurosurgeons in countries is not available but, as reported by some respondents, the majority are concentrated in urban areas.

◆ Implications

◆ Neurosurgeons complement the services provided by neurologists, most importantly to provide surgical services for neurological conditions. They provide expert care at secondary and tertiary level for neurosurgical emergencies such as head trauma and haemorrhage and also surgical care for conditions such as space-occupying lesions. In some places, neurosurgeons also provide medical care for people with neurological disorders. They also provide training, support and supervision to primary health-care providers in care of neurological conditions, especially emergencies.

◆ Training of general surgeons in neurosurgical emergencies is important in settings where it is not possible to have enough neurosurgeons at primary and secondary levels.

◆ The inequity in the number of neurosurgeons observed in countries in different income groups, population categories and geographical areas needs to be specifically studied and tackled.

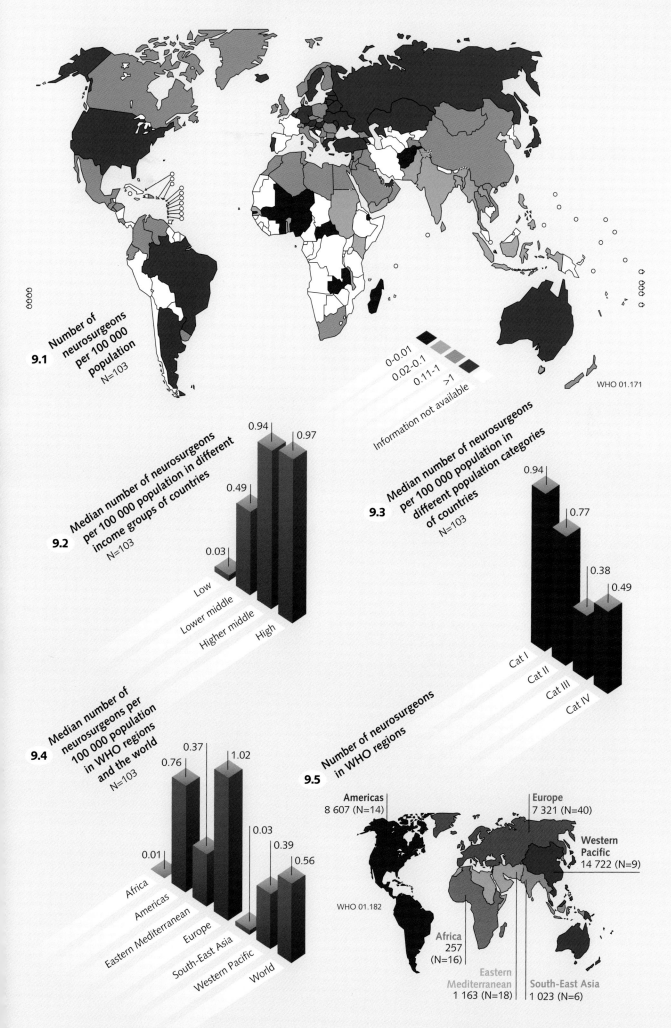

9.1 Number of neurosurgeons per 100 000 population
N=103

0-0.01
0.02-0.1
0.11-1
>1
Information not available

WHO 01.171

9.2 Median number of neurosurgeons per 100 000 population in different income groups of countries
N=103

0.03 — Low
0.49 — Lower middle
0.94 — Higher middle
0.97 — High

9.3 Median number of neurosurgeons per 100 000 population in different population categories of countries
N=103

0.94 — Cat I
0.77 — Cat II
0.38 — Cat III
0.49 — Cat IV

9.4 Median number of neurosurgeons per 100 000 population in WHO regions and the world
N=103

0.01 — Africa
0.76 — Americas
0.37 — Eastern Mediterranean
1.02 — Europe
0.03 — South-East Asia
0.39 — Western Pacific
0.56 — World

9.5 Number of neurosurgeons in WHO regions

Americas
8 607 (N=14)

Europe
7 321 (N=40)

Western Pacific
14 722 (N=9)

Africa
257 (N=16)

Eastern Mediterranean
1 163 (N=18)

South-East Asia
1 023 (N=6)

WHO 01.182

Neurology Atlas © 2004 WHO   33

◆ Definitions

- A **neuropaediatrician** is a specialist (neurologist or paediatrician) who has at least one year of recognized subspecialist training in child neurology.

◆ Salient Findings

- A total of 5733 neuropaediatricians are reported to be available in 98 countries. The median number of neuropaediatricians in the responding countries per 100 000 population is 0.10 (interquartile range 0.01–0.42). Since neuropaediatricians are specialists catering only for children, the median number of neuropaediatricians in the responding countries per 100 000 under-18 population is 0.33 (interquartile range 0.02–1.55).

- The median number of neuropaediatricians per 100 000 population varies widely across regions. It is 0 in Africa, 0.003 in South-East Asia, 0.06 in the Eastern Mediterranean, 0.08 in the Western Pacific, 0.12 in the Americas, and 0.47 in Europe. The median number of neuropaediatricians in the responding countries per 100 000 under-18 population is 0 in Africa, 0.007 in South-East Asia, 0.06 in the Eastern Mediterranean, 0.25 in the Americas, 0.26 in the Western Pacific, and 2.07 in Europe.

- Of the responding countries, 87.8% have less than one neuropaediatrician per 100 000 population. In fact, 23.5% of the responding countries do not have any neuropediatricians. In terms of population covered, more than one neuropaediatrician per 100 000 population is available for only 2.4% of the population.

- The median number of neuropaediatricians per 100 000 population across different income groups of countries also varies. It is 0.002 for low-income countries, compared to 0.25 for high-income countries.

- Even among high-income countries, only 7.7% of them have access to more than one neuropaediatrician per 100 000 population.

- The median number of neuropaediatricians is higher for countries with smaller populations (0.24 for countries in population category I) compared with 0.01 for countries in population category IV.

◆ Limitations

- In many countries, neuropaediatrics as a specialty does not exist; children with neurological problems are seen by neurologists or paediatricians with a special interest in neurology. This is true not only for developing countries but also for some developed ones.

- In some countries children with neurological disorders are also seen by child psychiatrists, and these are not included.

- Because the source of information in most of the countries was the national association of neurologists, it is possible that the neuropaediatricians who are not members of these associations were not included.

- In countries where neuropaediatricians exist, information about their distribution is not available. It is possible that the majority of them are concentrated in urban areas.

◆ Implications

- Children form a large proportion (40% or more in many countries) of the total population. Certain neurological disorders are also unique to children. Neuropaediatricians are therefore required at the tertiary level to provide specialist care. They are also needed to provide training, support and supervision to primary health-care providers involved in the neurological care of children.

- The inequity in the number of neuropaediatricians observed across income groups, population categories and geographical areas needs to be specifically studied and tackled. Often the regions with the lowest resources are those with the greatest proportions of children and no neuropaediatricians.

- It is also important to build the capacity of paediatricians who have a special interest in neurology so that they can manage neurological diseases more effectively.

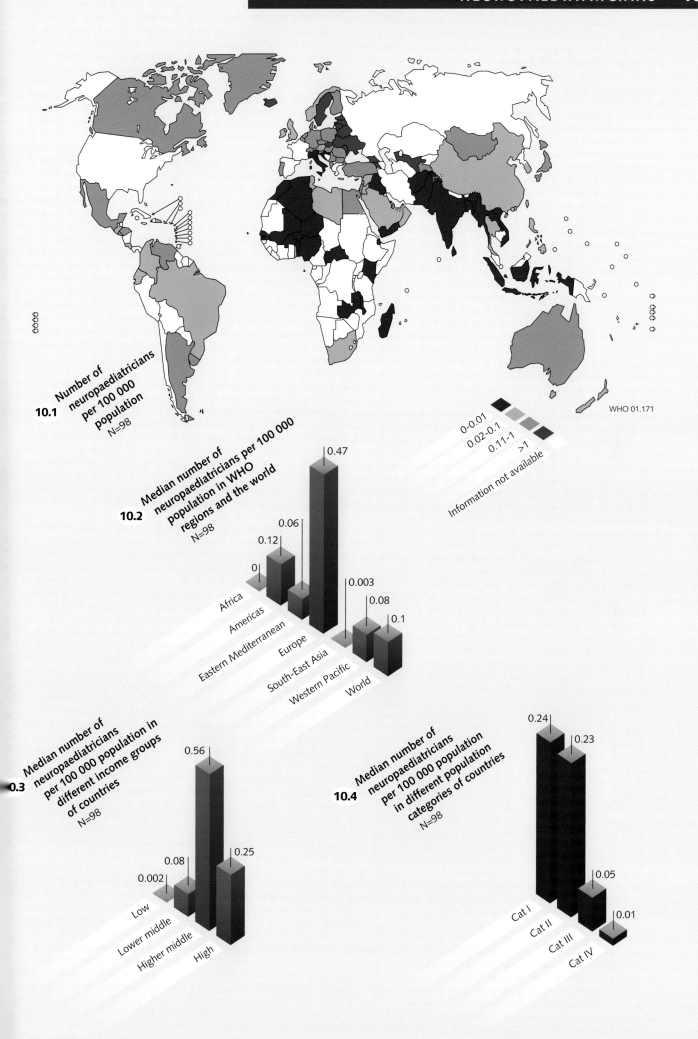

10.1 Number of neuropaediatricians per 100 000 population
N=98

WHO 01.171

0-0.01
0.02-0.1
0.11-1
>1
Information not available

10.2 Median number of neuropaediatricians per 100 000 population in WHO regions and the world
N=98

0.47
0.12
0.06
0
0.003
0.08
0.1

Africa
Americas
Eastern Mediterranean
Europe
South-East Asia
Western Pacific
World

0.3 Median number of neuropaediatricians per 100 000 population in different income groups of countries
N=98

0.56
0.002
0.08
0.25

Low
Lower middle
Higher middle
High

10.4 Median number of neuropaediatricians per 100 000 population in different population categories of countries
N=98

0.24
0.23
0.05
0.01

Cat I
Cat II
Cat III
Cat IV

◆ Definitions

- This theme refers to **postgraduate specialist training in neurology** for medical graduates from a recognized institution.

◆ Salient Findings

- Postgraduate training facilities in neurology are available in 76.2% of the responding countries. No facility for postgraduate training in neurology exists in 51.7% of low-income countries.

- Regionally, facilities for postgraduate training in neurology are variable. They exist in 31.3% of the responding countries in Africa and 47.4% in the Eastern Mediterranean. The facilities for postgraduate training are present in 88.9% of the responding countries in the Western Pacific, 92.9% in the Americas, 93% in Europe, and 100% in South-East Asia.

- The mean duration of training in neurology is 4.19 years (Standard Deviation (SD) 1.20). While the mean duration of training in neurology in low-income countries is 3.5 years (SD 1.3), it is 5.0 (SD 1.0) in high-income countries.

- A median number of 12 (interquartile range 5–30) students obtain a specialist degree in neurology every year in the responding countries. However, the median number of students obtaining a specialist degree in neurology every year per 100 000 population is 0.04 (interquartile range 0–0.19).

- The number of postgraduate students obtaining a specialist neurology degree per year per 100 000 population varies across different income groups of countries. The median number is 0 in low-income countries, while it is 0.15 in high-income countries.

- Regionally, the median number of postgraduate students obtaining a specialist degree in neurology per 100 000 population also varies. It is 0 in both Africa and the Eastern Mediterranean, 0.01 in South-East Asia, 0.04 in the Americas, 0.08 in the Western Pacific, and 0.20 in Europe.

- In 67.9% of the responding countries, students join postgraduate courses in neurology directly after medical graduation; in the rest, they join after a postgraduate course in internal medicine. Even in countries where students join postgraduate courses in neurology directly after medical graduation, some training in internal medicine is included in the neurology course.

◆ Limitations

- Data regarding the structure of training or the training curriculum are not available.

- Many countries send medical personnel abroad for training in neurology. Some of these graduates do not return to their countries of origin. The figures on trained specialists, therefore, may not reflect the number of specialists who remain available to work in the country.

- Within regions also, specialists trained in one country may go and work in other countries.

- Data regarding the content of neurology courses provided in medical undergraduate and internal medicine postgraduate training curricula was not obtained.

◆ Implications

- Education in the field of neurology is important for the continuous improvement of the delivery of neurological care. Although training facilities are available in a large number of countries, the number of postgraduates who obtain a specialist degree is clearly inadequate.

- An important component of neurological training concerns "brain drain", where graduates sent abroad for training do not return to practise in their countries of origin.

- Postgraduate neurological training facilities may not be needed in some smaller countries because of the high cost of establishing training facilities and the small number of trained professionals required. All regions, however, should have adequate facilities.

- A neurologist trained abroad may find it difficult to work in the home country because of differences in the epidemiology of neurological diseases as well as the availability of facilities. Thus there is a need to establish relevant training centres.

- The training content also varies, with some countries offering a greater emphasis on internal medicine as graduates join only after a specialization in internal medicine.

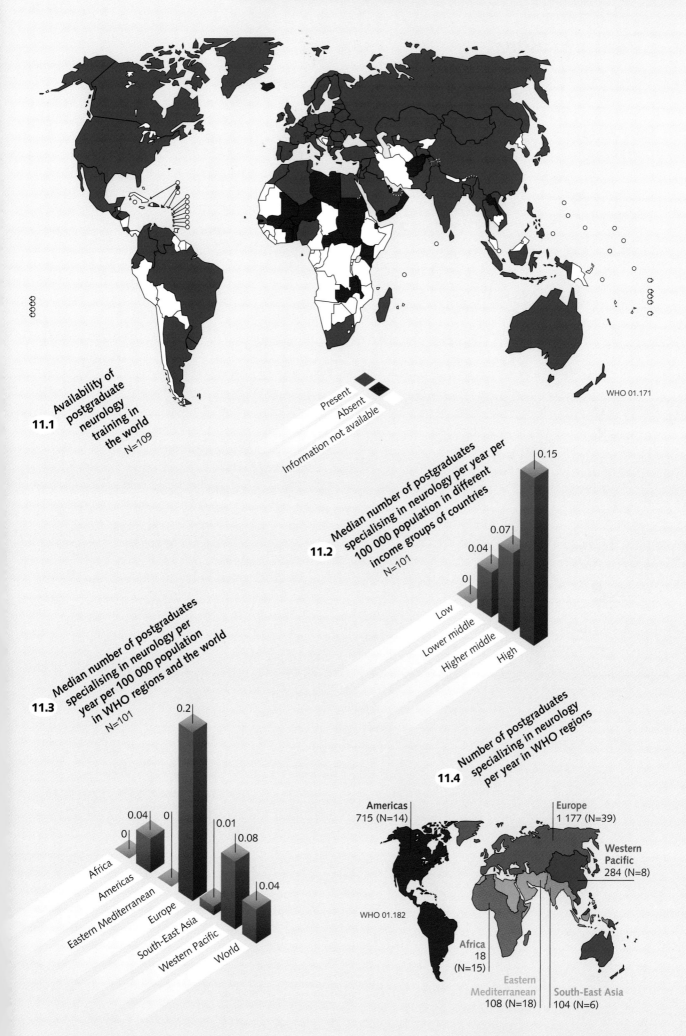

11.1 Availability of postgraduate neurology training in the world
N=109

Present
Absent
Information not available

WHO 01.171

11.2 Median number of postgraduates specialising in neurology per year per 100 000 population in different income groups of countries
N=101

0.15
0.07
0.04
0

Low
Lower middle
Higher middle
High

11.3 Median number of postgraduates specialising in neurology per year per 100 000 population in WHO regions and the world
N=101

0.2
0.04
0
0.04
0.01
0.08
0.04

Africa
Americas
Eastern Mediterranean
Europe
South-East Asia
Western Pacific
World

11.4 Number of postgraduates specializing in neurology per year in WHO regions

Americas
715 (N=14)

Europe
1 177 (N=39)

Western Pacific
284 (N=8)

Africa
18 (N=15)

Eastern Mediterranean
108 (N=18)

South-East Asia
104 (N=6)

WHO 01.182

◆ Definitions

- **Budget for neurological care** is defined as a separate regular source of money, available in a country's health budget allocated for actions directed towards the care of neurological disorders in the country.

- **Out-of-pocket payments** in this context refer to payments made for neurological care by the patient or his or her family.

- **Tax-based funding** refers to money for health services raised by general taxation or through taxes earmarked specifically for neurological services.

- **Social insurance** refers to a fixed percentage of income that everyone above a certain level of income is required to pay to a government-administered health insurance fund which, in return, pays for part or all of consumers' services for neurological care.

- **Private insurance** refers to a premium that health-care consumers pay voluntarily to a private insurance company which, in return, pays for part or all of their neurological care.

◆ Salient Findings

- Of the responding countries, 10.4% have a separate budget within the country's health budget for care of neurological illnesses.

- Tax-based funding and social insurance are the primary methods of financing neurological care in 37.8% and 35.4% of the responding countries, respectively, followed by out-of-pocket expenses in 25.6%. Private insurance is the primary method of financing in 1.2% of the responding countries.

- Out-of-pocket expenses are the most important source of financing in Africa (83.3% of the responding countries) and South-East Asia (40% of the responding countries).

- Tax-based funding is the most important source of financing in the Eastern Mediterranean (57.1% of the respond-

ing countries), the Western Pacific (50%), the Americas (42.9%) and South-East Asia (40%).

- Social insurance is the most important source of financing in Europe (58.3% of the responding countries), while none of the responding countries in Africa use social insurance as the primary method of financing.

- Out-of-pocket expenditure is the primary method of financing in 84.2% of low-income countries, while it is the primary method of financing in 3.6% of high-income countries.

- Tax-based funding and social insurance are primary methods of financing in 50% and 42.8% of high-income countries, respectively, and primary methods of financing in 10.5% and 5.3% of low-income countries, respectively.

◆ Limitations

- This information is based on best estimates by the respondents and not on a review of actual expenditure or budget figures.

- Although definitions were provided with the questionnaire, it is possible that they may not have been used accurately.

◆ Implications

- Although a separate budget for neurological services is not essential, when present it assists in earmarking the resources and planning the services effectively. In most countries, the budget for care of neurological diseases is included in somatic medicine.

- In most low-income countries, out-of-pocket payment is the major source of financing. This is likely to result in further inequity in utilization of neurological services. Efforts need to be made to introduce some form of public financing to cover these services.

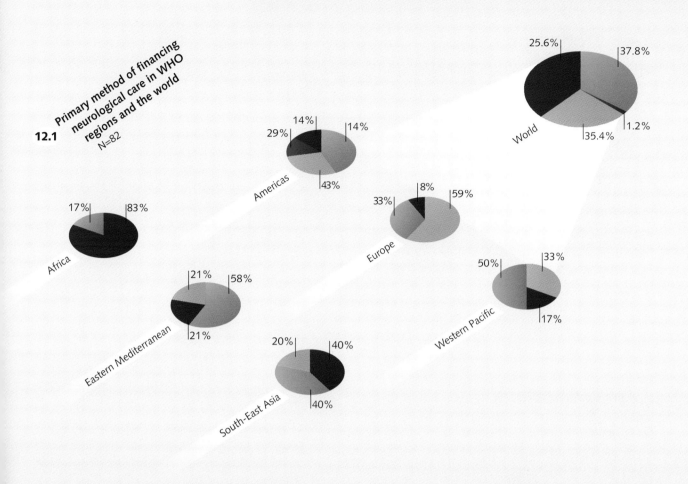

12.1 Primary method of financing neurological care in WHO regions and the world
N=82

World: 25.6%, 37.8%, 1.2%, 35.4%

Americas: 14%, 14%, 43%, 29%

Europe: 8%, 59%, 33%

Africa: 17%, 83%

Western Pacific: 33%, 17%, 50%

Eastern Mediterranean: 21%, 58%, 21%

South-East Asia: 20%, 40%, 40%

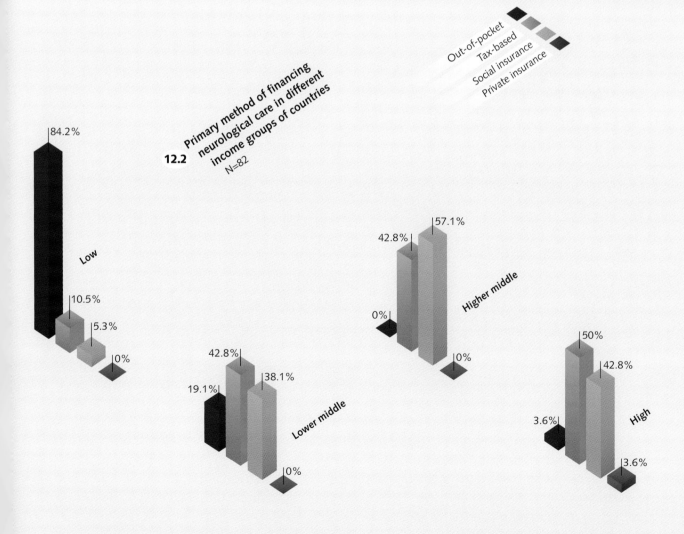

12.2 Primary method of financing neurological care in different income groups of countries
N=82

Out-of-pocket
Tax-based
Social insurance
Private insurance

Low: 84.2%, 10.5%, 5.3%, 0%

Lower middle: 19.1%, 42.8%, 38.1%, 0%

Higher middle: 0%, 42.8%, 57.1%, 0%

High: 3.6%, 50%, 42.8%, 3.6%

◆ Definitions

◆ **Disability benefits** in this context are the benefits that are payable as part of legal right from public funds in cases of neurological disorders that cause physical or mental impairment leading to functional limitations.

◆ Salient Findings

◆ Of the responding countries, 70.5% reported the availability of some form of disability benefits for patients with neurological disorders.

◆ Of the low-income countries, 67.9% reported nonavailability of any kind of disability benefit for neurological disorders, compared with 3.2% of high-income countries.

◆ Availability of disability benefits for neurological disorders is also variable across regions. While 25% and 33.3% of the responding countries in Africa and South-East Asia, respectively, reported availability of some form of disability benefits for neurological disorders, such benefits were available in 66.7% of the responding countries in the Eastern Mediterranean, 77.8% in the Western Pacific, 85.4% in Europe, and 92.3% in the Americas.

◆ Regarding the types of disability benefits reported by countries, monetary benefits (75.7%) and rehabilitation and health benefits (64.9%) are the most commonly reported, followed by other benefits including housing, transport, education and special discounts (45.9%) and benefits at the workplace (37.8%).

◆ Limitations

◆ Information on the exact type of disability benefit for neurological disorders was not obtained on a structured format.

◆ Data regarding coverage within the countries was not obtained. It is possible that in countries who responded in affirmative, disability benefits are available to only a small proportion of the population.

◆ Implications

◆ Because of a lack of public information about disability benefits and the procedure for claiming them, few people actually receive them in many countries even when benefits are available. Sometimes the procedure for availing themselves of disability benefits is also very complicated.

◆ Efforts should be made to advocate better provision of disability benefits for neurological disorders.

◆ The inequity in the availability of disability benefits observed across income groups, geographical areas and within countries needs to be specifically addressed.

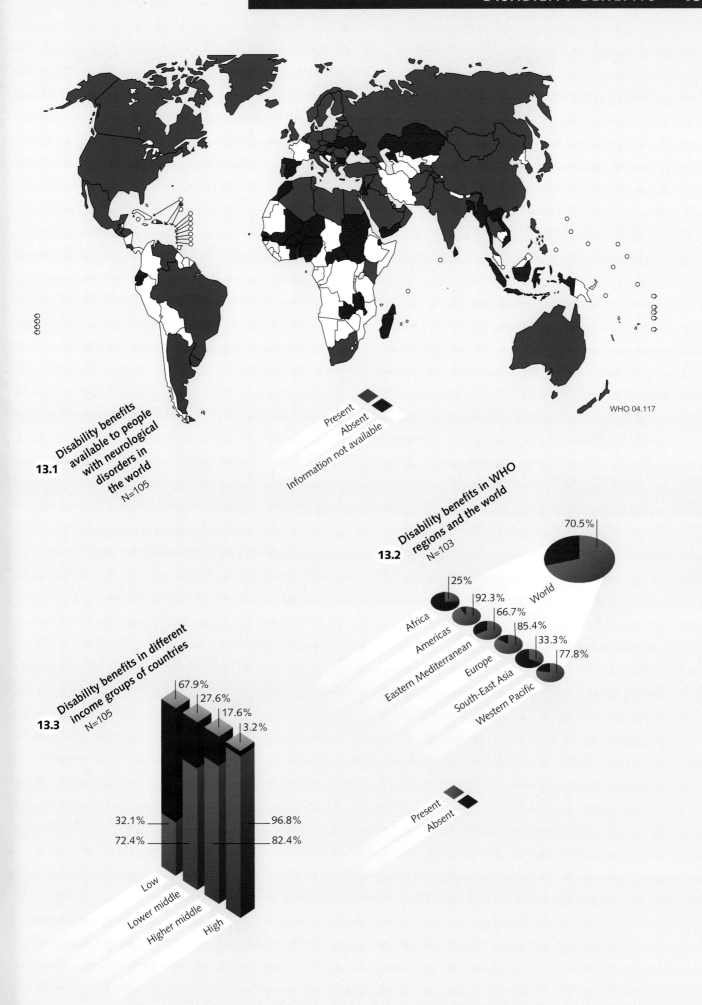

13.1 Disability benefits available to people with neurological disorders in the world
N=105

Present
Absent
Information not available

WHO 04.117

13.2 Disability benefits in WHO regions and the world
N=103

70.5% World
25% Africa
92.3% Americas
66.7% Eastern Mediterranean
85.4% Europe
33.3% South-East Asia
77.8% Western Pacific

13.3 Disability benefits in different income groups of countries
N=105

67.9%
27.6%
17.6%
3.2%

32.1% — — 96.8%
72.4% — — 82.4%

Low
Lower middle
Higher middle
High

Present
Absent

◆ Definitions

◆ In this context, **health reporting system** refers to the preparation of reports, usually yearly, covering health service functions related to neurological disorders, including the use of allocated funds.

◆ **Epidemiological or service data collection system** refers to an organized information-gathering system for service activity data for neurological disorders. It usually incorporates incidence and prevalence rates of diseases, admission and discharge rates, numbers of outpatient and community contacts and other activities.

◆ Salient Findings

◆ There is a health reporting system for neurological disorders in 78.1% of the responding countries.

◆ A health reporting system for neurological disorders is available in 66.7% and 73.3% of the responding countries in South-East Asia and Africa, respectively, while such a system is available in 76.9% of the responding countries in the Americas, 77.8% in the Eastern Mediterranean and the Western Pacific, and 83.3% in Europe.

◆ A data collection system for neurological disorders exists in 48.5% of the responding countries.

◆ Whereas almost two thirds of the responding countries in the Americas and Europe, 41.2% in the Eastern Mediterranean, and 43.8% in Africa have a data collection system for neurological disorders, none of the responding countries in South-East Asia and 22.2% in the Western Pacific have an epidemiological data collection system.

◆ An epidemiological data collection system is available in 35.7% of the low-income countries and 73.3% and 51.6% of the higher middle-income and high-income countries, respectively.

◆ Limitations

◆ Information about the quality or adequacy of the health reporting system for neurological disorders is not available.

◆ The epidemiological or service data collection system does not include the epidemiological studies for neurological disorders carried out by individual groups in various countries.

◆ Implications

◆ An organized health reporting system is essential to enable health planners to decide how to use various resources.

◆ Epidemiological data help to gather information regarding the disease burden and trends and help in identifying the high priority issues. This information is highly useful for planning health services and monitoring trends over time.

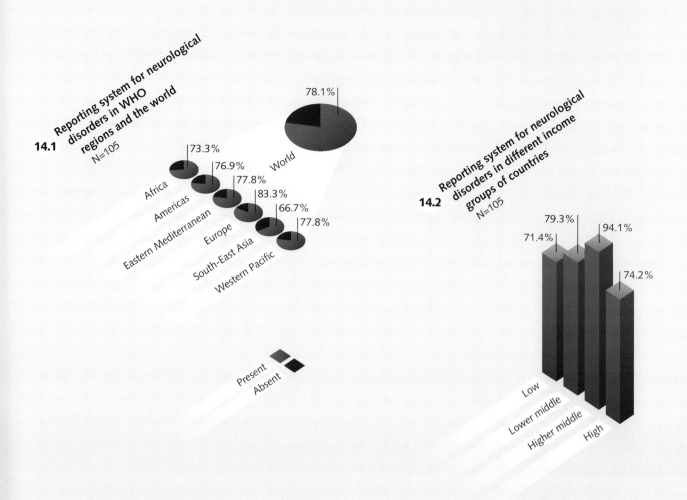

14.1 Reporting system for neurological disorders in WHO regions and the world
N=105

78.1% World

73.3% Africa
76.9% Americas
77.8% Eastern Mediterranean
83.3% Europe
66.7% South-East Asia
77.8% Western Pacific

Present
Absent

14.2 Reporting system for neurological disorders in different income groups of countries
N=105

71.4% Low
79.3% Lower middle
94.1% Higher middle
74.2% High

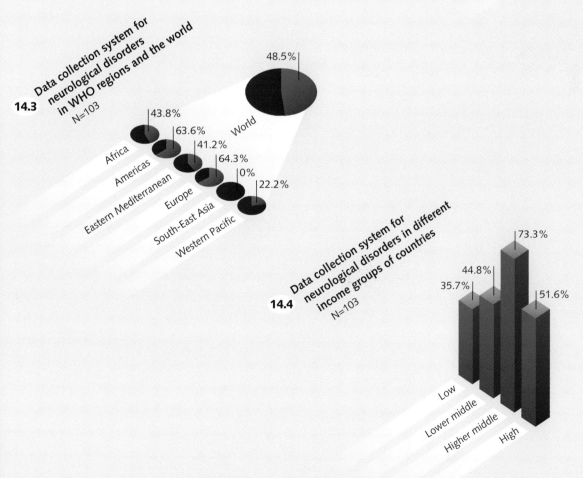

14.3 Data collection system for neurological disorders in WHO regions and the world
N=103

48.5% World

43.8% Africa
63.6% Americas
41.2% Eastern Mediterranean
64.3% Europe
0% South-East Asia
22.2% Western Pacific

14.4 Data collection system for neurological disorders in different income groups of countries
N=103

35.7% Low
44.8% Lower middle
73.3% Higher middle
51.6% High

◆ Definitions

◆ **National neurological association** refers to the professional association of neurologists or other neurology-allied sciences; such associations are usually nongovernmental.

◆ **Nongovernmental organizations (NGOs)** refers to voluntary organizations, charitable groups, service-user or advocacy groups in the area of neurology.

◆ Salient Findings

◆ A national neurological association exists in 87% of the responding countries.

◆ While 43.7% of the responding countries in Africa do not have a national neurological association, 26.3% in the Eastern Mediterranean, 11.1% in the Western Pacific and 2.3% in Europe do not have a national neurological association.

◆ A median number of 192 (interquartile range 46–500) specialists are members of the national neurological association in the responding countries.

◆ The national neurological associations are involved in various activities: organizing professional meetings and conferences (100% of the responding countries), advising government (70.7%), constructing curricula for postgraduate training (44.6%), granting a degree of specialization in neurology (31.5%), constructing curricula for undergraduate training (30.4%), accrediting neurology departments for postgraduate training (28.3%) and accrediting neurology departments for undergraduate training (21.7%).

◆ Of the responding countries, 71.7% have at least one nongovernmental organization working in the field of neurology. In 10.5% of these countries, the nongovernmental organizations are working only in the area of epilepsy.

◆ No nongovernmental organizations for neurological disorders exist in 34% of the low-income countries and 29% of the high-income countries.

◆ Regionally, no nongovernmental organizations for neurological disorders exist in 52.9% of the responding countries in the Eastern Mediterranean, 33.3% in the Western Pacific, 23.8% in Europe, 19.7% in Africa, 16.7% in South-East Asia, and 14.3% in the Americas.

◆ The nongovernmental organizations are involved in awareness and advocacy in 92.1% of the responding countries, treatment (69.7%), rehabilitation (65.8%) and prevention (61.8%) activities.

◆ Limitations

◆ Since the sources of information in most countries were the key persons working in neurology and possibly members of a national association, the data pertain mainly to countries where neurologists or persons with an interest in neurology exist. Therefore it is possible that the figures might be an overestimate.

◆ Information regarding the coverage of population by the activities specified within the countries is not available.

◆ Information regarding the quality of services is also lacking.

◆ Some of the nongovernmental organizations working in the countries are actually international organizations and not local organizations.

◆ Implications

◆ Presence of professional associations highlights the commitment of neurologists to improve the status of care for neurological disorders.

◆ The neurological associations should be more involved to improve the status of patient care and training in neurology.

◆ The participation of both local as well as international nongovernmental organizations in the care of neurological disorders is important. Their activities need to be encouraged as they complement the services provided by the public sector.

◆ Many international nongovernmental organizations are also involved in various educational and training activities for neurologists.

◆ Groups of patients with neurological disorders and their carers need to be established in many more countries, as they can be strong advocates for improvement in the quality of services.

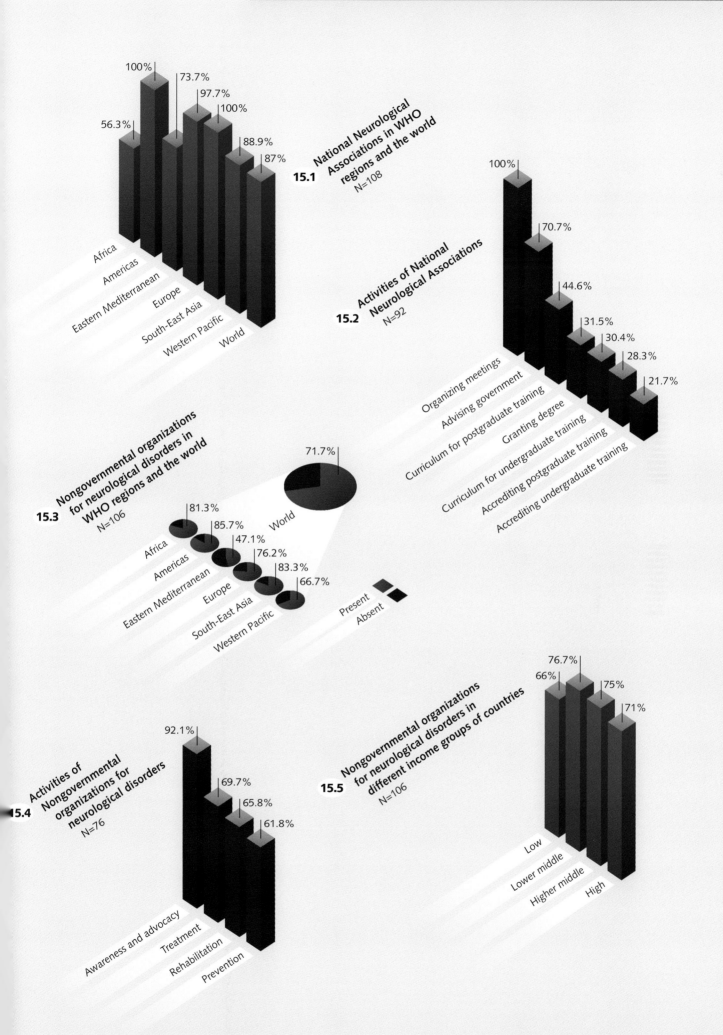

15.1 National Neurological Associations in WHO regions and the world
N=108

Africa 56.3%
Americas 100%
Eastern Mediterranean 73.7%
Europe 97.7%
South-East Asia 100%
Western Pacific 88.9%
World 87%

15.2 Activities of National Neurological Associations
N=92

Organizing meetings 100%
Advising government 70.7%
Curriculum for postgraduate training 44.6%
Granting degree 31.5%
Curriculum for undergraduate training 30.4%
Accrediting postgraduate training 28.3%
Accrediting undergraduate training 21.7%

15.3 Nongovernmental organizations for neurological disorders in WHO regions and the world
N=106

World 71.7%
Africa 81.3%
Americas 85.7%
Eastern Mediterranean 47.1%
Europe 76.2%
South-East Asia 83.3%
Western Pacific 66.7%

Present
Absent

15.4 Activities of Nongovernmental organizations for neurological disorders
N=76

Awareness and advocacy 92.1%
Treatment 69.7%
Rehabilitation 65.8%
Prevention 61.8%

15.5 Nongovernmental organizations for neurological disorders in different income groups of countries
N=106

Low 66%
Lower middle 76.7%
Higher middle 75%
High 71%

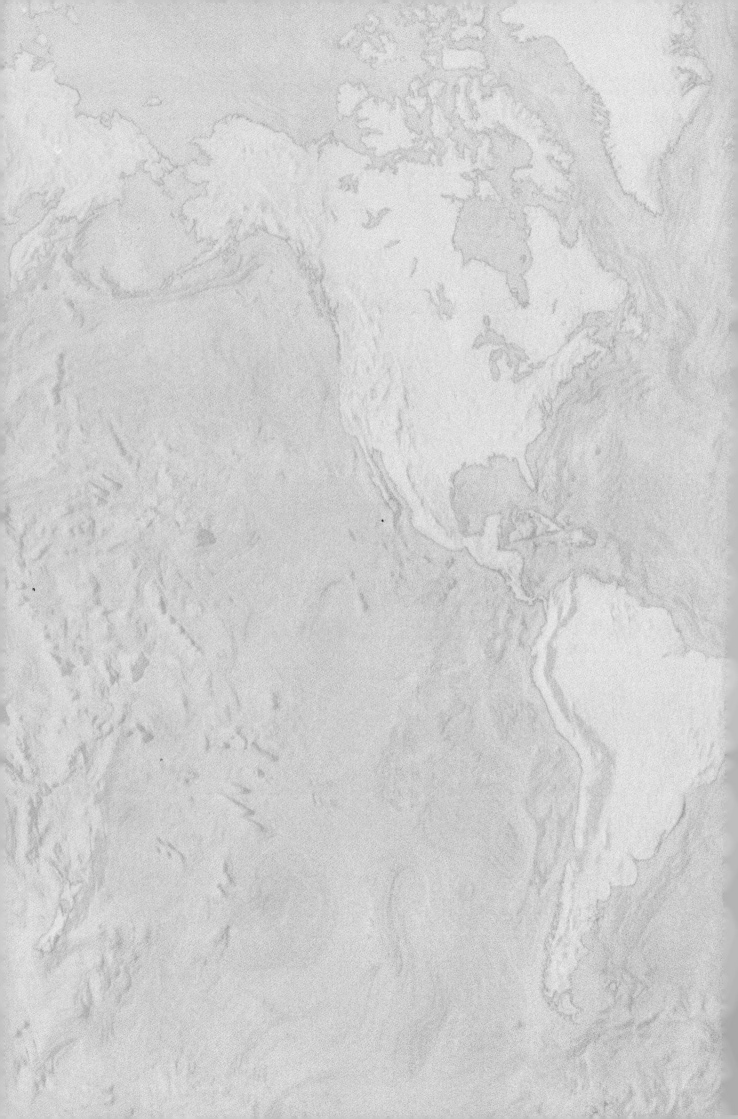

The following pages provide a focus on selected areas in relation to neurology. The specialists who contributed the reviews are listed in the Project Team and Partners.

Epilepsy is one of the most common serious disorders of the brain, affecting some 50 million people worldwide. It is unique among these disorders in that its symptoms can be completely controlled in the majority of affected individuals by inexpensive medications or cost-effective surgical procedures, and many forms of epilepsy can be prevented by appropriate public health interventions. Epilepsy accounts for 1% of the global burden of disease, determined by the number of productive life-years lost as a result of disability or premature death (50). Among primary disorders of the brain, this burden ranks with depression and other affective disorders, Alzheimer's disease and other dementias, and substance abuse; among all medical conditions, it ranks with breast cancer in women and lung cancer in men.

Approximately one in 10 people can expect to have at least one epileptic seizure during a normal lifespan, but one seizure is not epilepsy. Only a third of the people who experience a seizure have an enduring brain disturbance that causes recurrent seizures and therefore warrants a diagnosis of epilepsy. Despite epilepsy being so common, the reported figures vary widely. The incidence is generally taken to be between 40 and 70 per 100 000 people per year in industrialized countries, with estimates of 100–190 per 100 000 people per year in developing countries (51, 52). The prevalence is between 5 and 40 per 1000 persons (51). Parasitic, viral and bacterial infections have been suggested as important factors in the cause of epilepsy in developing countries (52). Other important causes include brain damage at birth caused by asphyxia, infections, and brain trauma resulting from accidents. Some of the public health policies which may help in modifying these risk factors include better perinatal care, strategies to control head injury, better hygiene to decrease neurocysticercosis, and immunization. In the affluent countries, reduction of stroke by modifying the risk factors may lessen the incidence of epilepsy.

Evidence exists that 60–70% of people with epilepsy could lead normal lives if properly treated with antiepileptic drugs (AEDs) (53). Some of them will need to continue with medication for life but, for others, the antiepileptic medication may eventually be stopped without seizures recurring. For some patients with intractable epilepsy, neurosurgical treatment may be successful.

Of the burden of epilepsy worldwide, 80% is in the developing world, where 80% of people with epilepsy receive no treatment at all (52). In most of these regions, misconceptions, stigma, and discrimination are greater obstacles to the well-being of people with epilepsy than lack of adequate health-care facilities. These problems can be solved relatively inexpensively through education of patients, their families, the general public, health-care providers and government agencies, as well as through improved access to effective treatments. A Global Campaign Against Epilepsy, a joint effort of the International League against Epilepsy (ILAE), the International Bureau for Epilepsy (IBE) and WHO, is currently in progress in order to reduce the treatment gap for epilepsy and promote acceptance of people with this disorder by bringing epilepsy "out of the shadows" (54). The aim of the Campaign is to provide better information about epilepsy and its consequences and to assist governments and those concerned with epilepsy to reduce the burden of the disorder.

Much more basic and clinical research is necessary to develop new approaches for prevention, diagnosis, and treatment, and to devise cost-effective ways to bring currently available approaches to the developing areas of the world where limited resources and tropical conditions remain a major obstacle to adequate health care.

Stroke is the second leading cause of death after ischemic heart disease worldwide, with an estimated 5.5 million subjects dying from stroke every year. Two thirds of these deaths occur in countries with low resources. Approximately 80% of patients survive the acute phase of stroke: 50–75% of the survivors are left with varying degrees of chronic disability, thus making stroke a leading cause of disability in adults.

Hospital care, long-term care, complete or partial working incapacity, and community support – all of these factors cause enormous costs for the patients, their families, communities and the health-care system. There are different estimates of costs of management of stroke per patient in various regions. In Australia, the European Union and North America, the mean total cost of stroke management for the first three months is approximately US$ 14 000. The average cost per surviving day is US$ 260 (55). In general, more than 70% of costs are directed for covering hospitalization, less than 20% for rehabilitation, and the rest for chronic care facilities. Lifetime costs per stroke patient range approximately between US$ 60 000 and US$ 230 000. These costs should be regarded in the context of the epidemiological data, as the number of stroke survivors in a society translates directly into the actual economic burden of stroke.

Surveys performed before 1990 show that the worldwide crude prevalence rate of stroke in all age groups ranges from 4 to 20 per 1000 population. More recently published data from population-based studies show less variability between geographical regions, with the crude prevalence rate ranging from 5 to 10 per 1000 population (56). Some gender differences can be observed, as the stroke prevalence rate is lower in women than in men. Despite the stable rates, demographic estimates point towards an important increase of the number of strokes in the near future – especially in South America and Asia.

Based on these simple data one can roughly estimate the life-time costs of all strokes as millions of dollars in a medium-sized European country, thus highlighting the importance of stroke as a target for public health campaigns. However, stroke-related costs should not be regarded from a perspective of a high-income country. With the increasing burden of stroke in low-income countries the same magnitude of resources would be required to fulfil the needs of patients and to cover the disability-related loss of productivity.

As prevention is more effective than treatment, primary health care is the most appropriate means of preventing stroke and reducing its public health impact. It is crucial to increase awareness among primary care physicians of modifiable stroke risk factors such as hypertension, diabetes mellitus, tobacco smoking, obesity and excessive alcohol consumption. This knowledge will allow for institution of primary and secondary prevention measures. It is also of great importance to introduce stroke awareness campaigns for the public, to promote healthy lifestyles and demonstrate the need for risk factor modification. Stroke should be regarded as one of the preventable cardiovascular diseases, and stroke prevention should be a global effort.

Data from the literature shows that organized care in a stroke unit is the most effective way of reducing long-term case fatality, long-term disability and the need for institutionalization (57). The benefits of a stroke unit come from its focus on coordinated multidisciplinary care, nursing integration and early rehabilitation. Specialization of care represented by interest and expertise in stroke rehabilitation, and also education and training of staff, patients and caregivers, are of great importance. Efforts need to be made to popularize and promote stroke unit care, especially in countries with low and medium levels of resources.

Important endeavours have been undertaken recently to improve the knowledge of stroke epidemiology worldwide. The Surveillance and Risk Assessment Division of the Population and Public Health Branch of Health, Canada – a WHO Collaborating Centre for Surveillance of Cardiovascular Diseases – developed a database of worldwide demographic data on cardiovascular and cerebrovascular disease mortality and morbidity. Moreover, the World Federation of Neurology and the International Stroke Society, in collaboration with WHO, have initiated the development of a stroke component of the WHO Global Noncommunicable Disease Infobase, which collects information on stroke prevalence, incidence, mortality and case fatality based on published data. Another WHO-initiated activity is an international stroke surveillance system: the STEPwise approach, which will form a framework for surveillance and data collection in order to achieve comparability of data over time and between different countries (58, 59). All these efforts aim to improve prevention and control of stroke and to facilitate the planning of health services. A joint effort of health-care professionals, nongovernmental organizations and governmental bodies is the key to controlling epidemics of stroke.

Headache disorders are ubiquitous. Their lifetime prevalence in populations in which they have been measured is over 90%. Migraine is most studied, although still not fully in all regions of the world. It mostly affects people of working age but does trouble children as well. European and American studies show that 6–8% of men and 15–18% of women experience migraine every year (60). A similar pattern is seen in Central and South America: in Puerto Rico, for example, 6% of men and 17% of women are affected. Major studies are still to be conducted in India, but anecdotal evidence suggests similar levels of migraine promoted by Indian lifestyle factors. In Japan it is estimated to affect 8.4% of adults. Migraine appears less prevalent, but still common, elsewhere in Asia (3% of men and 10% of women) and in Africa (3–7% in community-based studies). Again in these areas, major studies have yet to be conducted. The higher rates in women everywhere (2–3 times those in men) are hormonally driven.

Tension-type headache (TTH) is the most common headache disorder (61). Most is episodic, and this subtype affects two-thirds of adult males and over 80% of females in developed countries, although few seriously. In its chronic subtype, in contrast, it is present on more days than not and is disabling. Chronic tension-type headache overlaps with and is sometimes indistinguishable from other forms of chronic daily headache, some of which are unrelentingly present throughout every day. Estimates of the prevalence of this group of conditions in Europe and the United States are as high as 1 in 25 of the adult population (62).

Not only is headache painful but, depending on its intensity and other symptoms that may accompany it, it is also disabling. Migraine affects people particularly during their productive years and, in a survey in the United States, 80% of people with migraine reported disability because of it. Extrapolation from migraine prevalence and attack incidence data suggests that 3000 migraine attacks occur every day for each million of the general population so it is unsurprising that, worldwide, migraine is 19th among all causes of years of life lost to disability (YLDs) (63). As well as suffering directly from its symptoms, people with migraine consistently score highly on scales of general physical and mental ill-health. Chronic tension-type headache and other forms of chronic daily headache are associated with long-term morbidity.

Repeated headache attacks, and often the constant fear of the next, damage family life, social life and employment. For example, social activity and work capacity are reduced in almost all migraine sufferers and in 60% of tension-type headache sufferers. The financial cost of headache arises partly from direct treatment costs but much more from loss of work-time and productivity. In the United Kingdom, for example, 25 million workdays or schooldays are lost every year because of migraine alone. A recent United States study measured indirect costs in a managed-care population at over US$ 4500 per sufferer per year. Tension-type headache and chronic daily headache may together cause losses of similar magnitude. In the 15 European Union countries prior to enlargement, the annual cost of all headache has been estimated at € 10 000-30 000 million.

Therefore, while headache rarely signals serious underlying illness, it is high among causes of consulting both general practitioners and neurologists. Over a period of five years, one in six patients aged 16–65 years in a large general practice in the United Kingdom consulted because of headache. A survey of neurologists found that up to one third of all their patients consulted for headache – more than for any other single complaint.

Despite headache being a common occurrence, there is good evidence that large numbers of people troubled by it do not receive effective health care. In many countries, headache conditions are not recognized as diseases but only as self-limiting and unimportant symptoms, deserving no allocation at all of resources. A consensus conference organized by the American and International Headache Societies concluded that migraine is underdiagnosed and undertreated throughout the world.

Nevertheless there are effective treatments. It is possible to alleviate much of the symptom burden of headache and thereby mitigate both the humanitarian and the financial costs. Crucially, the common headache disorders require no special investigation and their diagnosis and management call only for skills generally available to physicians. Most headache can be optimally managed in primary care, if the following barriers are removed:

◆ lack of knowledge, among health-care providers, of headache disorders and how to treat them;

◆ poor awareness among the general public, so that headaches are often trivialized as a minor annoyance and an excuse to avoid responsibility (stigmatization), and among headache sufferers who are unaware that effective treatments exist;

◆ failure of governments to acknowledge the burden of headache and to recognize that the costs of treating it are small in comparison with the huge savings that might be made (for example, by reducing lost working days) if resources were allocated to do so appropriately.

The key to successful health care for headache in most areas of the world is therefore education. This is at the heart of the Global Campaign to Reduce the Burden of Headache (64).

Parkinson's disease occurs worldwide: it affects all ethnic groups and socioeconomic classes. Besides the disabling motor symptoms, patients have non-motor symptoms such as anxiety and depression. The Global Parkinson's disease Survey in six countries demonstrated that depression in Parkinson's disease is a significant factor affecting the health-related quality of life (65). Although there is no cure for Parkinson's disease, there have been advances in its management through drugs, rehabilitative measures and surgery. To achieve health for all, it is essential that we have a true appraisal of the epidemiological aspects of Parkinson's disease and resources available in each region.

Most epidemiological studies have shown an estimated incidence ranging from 16 to 19 per 100000 people per year (66), while estimated crude prevalence is 160 per 100000 people per year (67). There are regional variations which may, in part, be attributable to different methods of case-finding, diagnostic criteria and the age of the population. There is clearly a need for well-defined epidemiological studies, especially from the developing regions of the world.

Parkinson's disease poses a significant public health burden, which is likely to increase in the coming years. Along with other neurodegenerative diseases such as Alzheimer's disease, Parkinson's disease is expected to surpass cancer as the second most common cause of death by the year 2040. The direct and indirect costs for the care of Parkinsonian patients, including cost of drug treatment (about US$ 1100 million worldwide) can be substantial (68). The incidence and prevalence of Parkinson's disease increase with advancing age, occurring in about 1% of people over the age of 65 years. With increase in life expectancy, future demographic projections predict a larger population over the age of 60 years in the developing regions, with a corresponding increase in the number of Parkinson patients.

For delivery of neurological care to people with Parkinson's disease, adequate human resources and other facilities are required. These are regrettably deficient, especially in the developing regions. For instance, there are only about 850 neurologists for the care of over 1000 million people in India (1 neurologist for 1.2 million inhabitants). These neurologists are mainly located in the cities, whereas nearly two thirds of India's population reside in rural areas. It is therefore necessary to seek the help of primary care physicians for the care of patients. Medical education should be suitably modified so that graduate physicians are able to recognize primary symptoms of Parkinson's disease and impart education about this illness to patients and their families. They should be able to initiate treatment with the appropriate anti-Parkinsonian drug and refer suitable cases to community hospitals in semi-urban areas or to large urban hospitals. There is also a great need to expand the support services and to have more nurse specialists, social workers, paramedical staff and rehabilitation centres. Various nongovernmental support organizations are working in this area to increase the awareness of this disease and its management.

Dementia is a syndrome characterized by a progressive global deterioration in intellectual function. Alzheimer's disease is the commonest pathology, accounting for 50% to 75% of cases. Recent estimates for numbers of people with dementia worldwide suggest that 18–25 million persons were affected in 2000 and that this number will double to 32–40 million by 2020 (69, 70). It is largely a disease of older persons: only 2% of cases are under 65 years of age. After this age, the prevalence doubles with every five-year increment in age. Prevalence varies very little between developed countries: 1% for 60–64 years, 1.5% for 65–69 years, 3% for 70–74 years, 6% for 75–79 years, 13% for 80–84 years, 24% for 85–89 years, 34% for 90–94 years, and 45% for those aged 95 years or over (70).

Demographic ageing proceeds apace in China, India and Latin America. In the 30 years up to 2020, the oldest sector of the population will have increased by 200% in developing countries compared with 68% in the developed world (2). By 2020, two thirds of all people over 60 (and, presumably, a similar proportion of all those with dementia) will be living in developing countries (69). In the developing world, however, there is more uncertainty as to the frequency of dementia, with few studies and widely varying estimates (71). In general, prevalence and incidence are lower than in the developed countries (71). Early onset cases are again rare, though this may be changing in parts of the world where HIV/AIDS is endemic.

Dementia is one of the major causes of disability in later life. The consensus estimated disability weight for dementia applied in the global burden of disease report was higher than that for almost any other condition with the exception of spinal cord injury and terminal cancer. Among older people, dementia was the most burdensome neuropsychiatric disorder accounting for more than half of all disability-adjusted life years in this domain of morbidity (2).

People with dementia are heavy consumers of health services, but in developed countries most direct costs arise from community and residential care. In the United Kingdom these costs amount to US$ 8000 million, or US$ 13 000 per person with dementia (72). The economic burden is unevenly distributed; families from the poorest countries are particularly likely to use expensive private medical services and to be spending more than 10% of per capita GNP on health care (73). Worldwide, family caregivers are the cornerstone of support for people with dementia. They experience significant psychological, practical and economic strain (73, 74). Dementia care is particularly time intensive because of the need for close supervision. Many caregivers need to give up or cut back upon work in order to care. When the full costs of their care inputs were calculated, in the United States they amounted to US$ 18 000 million annually (75).

Primary prevention should probably focus upon risk factors for vascular disease, including hypertension, smoking, type II diabetes, and hyperlipidaemia. The epidemic of smoking in developing countries and the high and rising prevalence of type II diabetes in Asia are particular causes of concern. More work is needed to identify further modifiable risk factors.

Achieving progress with dementia care has much to do with creating the climate for change. Lack of awareness, widespread among policy-makers, clinicians and the general public, is a key public health problem with important consequences:

- affected persons do not seek help; even if they do, health-care services tend not to meet their needs;

- dementia is stigmatized; for example, sufferers can be excluded from residential care and denied admission to hospital facilities;

- there is no constituency to lobby government or policy-makers;

- families are the main caregivers, but they lack support or understanding from others.

Population level interventions are needed. National Alzheimer Associations help to raise awareness and create a framework for positive engagement between clinicians, researchers, caregivers and people with dementia.

Primary health-care services have an essential role to play in prevention, detection and management. Clinic-based services providing acute care do not meet this need. For many low-income countries the most cost-effective approach will be community primary care services supporting, educating and advising family caregivers, supplemented by subsidized home nursing or home-care workers. Day care and residential respite care are more expensive, but nevertheless basic to a community's needs, particularly for more advanced dementia. Residential care is unlikely to be a government priority. Even in some of the poorer countries, however, private nursing and residential care homes are opening to meet the new demand (for example, in China and India). If government policies are well formulated, the inevitable shift of resource expenditure towards older people can be predicted and its consequences mitigated (76).

Multiple sclerosis is the most common neurological disorder in younger adults of Caucasian origin. The etiology is still unknown but pathogenetic steps leading to the characteristic histological findings of perivascular inflammation and focal demyelination, as well as astrocyte scarring and axonal loss, have become better understood.

Clinically the disease course is most often relapsing-remitting, with exacerbations lasting on average a few weeks to a few months. In the long run, over decades, this course most often turns (for unknown reasons) into a secondary progression. The cases which remain relapsing-remitting are probably the ones which are benign (10–15%). Another form of the disease is primary progressive, equally frequent in females and males with probably less inflammatory components. In relapsing-remitting and secondary progressive forms the disease is twice as common in females than in males.

The world estimate is 1.11 to 2.5 million cases of multiple sclerosis. High-frequency zones for multiple sclerosis at 50–100 per 100 000 population are Europe, Canada, countries of the former USSR, Israel, northern United States, New Zealand, and south-east Australia. Lowest frequency zones for multiple sclerosis at 5 per 100 000 population are Asia, Africa and South America. In general, multiple sclerosis occurs worldwide with much greater frequency in higher latitudes between 40 and 60 degrees north and south latitude (77, 78).

As long as the etiology of multiple sclerosis remains unknown, a causal therapy or effective prevention is not possible. Introduction of new disease-modifying therapies such as beta-interferon or glatiramer acetate may alter the disease course, especially in the relapsing-remitting form, by reducing the number of attacks by about a third and reducing the accumulation of lesions as seen on MRI, and by influencing the impact of the disease on disability. Rehabilitation still remains the most effective element in the overall management of multiple sclerosis. Clinical as well as basic research are urgently needed in a coordinated fashion in order to find the etiology of this still enigmatic disease, with the goal of finding more effective treatments or preventing it altogether.

Most care for disorders of the nervous system is provided not by neurologists but by general physicians and other primary health-care workers, especially in developing countries where neurologists may be few or nonexistent. Adequate pregraduation training in neurology is needed everywhere so that general physicians can identify and treat disorders of the nervous system, which are major contributors to the global burden of disease.

Undergraduate medical curricula should include the epidemiology and prevention of the neurological disorders that are most prevalent in the region where graduates will practise. Some of the commonest neurological disorders such as stroke and epilepsy are preventable to some degree, for example by adequate treatment of hypertension in the first case and by eradication of neurocysticercosis in the other. The beneficial effects of neurorehabilitation and the careful management of chronic neurological diseases should also be included in pregraduate curricula.

To keep physicians abreast of changing patterns of neurological disorders (such as the increasing incidence of cerebrovascular disease and dementia in developing countries), continuing medical education in neurology should be readily available to all primary care physicians. Particularly in countries where neurospecialists are few, and most care of neurological disorders falls to the primary care physician or other health-care professionals, the educational role of the neurologist should include providing continuing medical education for primary care doctors (79). Continuing medical education for neurologists is widely available in wealthier countries through national and international neurological societies. For neurologists in developing countries, regional neurological societies can offer educational programmes that focus attention on neurological disorders endemic to the area, and foster connections with neurologists in wealthier countries.

Neurologists everywhere are recognized by their expertise in certain areas such as basic neurosciences, the neurological history and examination, and diagnosis and management of neurological disorders. Physicians in some countries may identify themselves as neurologists after minimal specialty training, whereas in other countries several years of postgraduate education, followed by successful completion of a specialty examination, are necessary. Through their national professional organizations, neurologists serve as advisers to national governments in over 70% of countries. Where this is the case, neurology curricula should also include some training in public health and in health-care delivery.

There are no recognized international standards for training in the specialty of neurology or for methods of demonstrating competency in the field. Postgraduate neurology curricula vary widely, some concentrating on clinical training and others stressing knowledge in basic neurosciences. Many of these differences spring naturally from local needs, and are not necessarily undesirable. There are wide regional differences in the prevalence of various neurological disorders. A core curriculum in neurology should be influenced by local conditions, particularly for training in neuroepidemiology, prevention of neurological disorders, changing patterns of disease, and the cost-effective use of diagnostic and therapeutic resources.

The length of training programmes in neurology varies from place to place. Areas of subspecialty training in neurology include stroke, movement disorders, epilepsy, neurorehabilitation, pain, and clinical neurophysiology, and such programmes are generally available only in the wealthiest countries. They usually require one to two years, but accurate data about the length and content of such programmes are lacking. Whether adequate neurology training might be done in less time in certain countries or regions would be a useful subject for study. Shorter programmes would be less costly and might require fewer faculty members.

The available data demonstrate that in many low-income and middle-income countries there may be no neurologists, or as few as one neurologist for every 2 million people (47). Such countries generally do not have the conventional academic foundations for postgraduate neurology training programmes, and their neurologists receive training elsewhere. For small countries, the model of specialty training abroad may be suitable, as long as the training corresponds to the disease profile and technological milieu of the country where the neurologist will practise. The establishment or improvement of neurology training programmes is desirable in larger countries, however, to produce graduates who will work locally or in the region. The organization and evaluation of new training programmes could be facilitated by international linkages with various nongovernmental organizations.

In some areas the construction of regional training programmes could avoid duplication of costly resources and allow pooling of resources. Modern technology would facilitate the use of long-distance teaching, sharing of teaching materials, and establishment of research ties. In some regions it might be desirable to replace or supplement the traditional four-year postgraduate neurology programme with a shorter training programme for general physicians with a special interest in clinical neurology.

1. *WHO – What it is, what it does*. Geneva, World Health Organization, 1988.

2. Murray CJL, Lopez AD, eds. *The global burden of disease: a comprehensive assessment of mortality and disability from diseases, injuries and risk factors in 1990 and projected to 2020*. Cambridge, MA, Harvard School of Public Health on behalf of the World Health Organization and the World Bank, 1996 (Global Burden of Disease and Injury Series, Vol. I).

3. *Atlas of mental health resources in the world*. Geneva, World Health Organization, 2001.

4. Janca A, Prilipko L, Saraceno B. Neurology and public health: a World Health Organization perspective. *Archives of Neurology*, 2000, 57:1786–1788.

5. *World Bank list of economies (July, 2003)*. Washington, DC, World Bank (http://www.worldbank.org, accessed February 2004).

6. *The world health report 2003 – Shaping the future*. Geneva, World Health Organization, 2003.

7. Murray TJ. Concepts in undergraduate neurological teaching. *Clinical Neurology and Neurosurgery*, 1976, 79:275–284.

8. Marsland DW, Wood M, Mayo F. The content of family practice. *Journal of Family Practice*, 1976, 3:23–74.

9. Miller JQ. The neurologic content of family practice. Implications for neurologists. *Archives of Neurology*, 1986, 43:286–288.

10. Hopkins A. Lessons for neurologists from the United Kingdom third national morbidity survey. *Journal of Neurology, Neurosurgery and Psychiatry*, 1989, 52:430–433.

11. Papapetropoulos T, Tsibre E, Pelekoudas V. The neurological content of general practice. *Journal of Neurology, Neurosurgery and Psychiatry*, 1989, 52:434–435.

12. van den Bosch JH, Kardaun JW. [Disease burden of nervous system disorders in the Netherlands]. *Nederlands Tijdschrift voor Geneeskunde*, 1994, 138:1219–1224.

13. Heckmann JG, Duran JC, Galeoto J. [The incidence of neurological disorders in tropical South America. Experience in the Bolivian lowlands]. *Fortschritte der Neurologie-Psychiatrie*, 1997, 65:291–296.

14. Birbeck GL. Barriers to care for patients with neurologic disease in rural Zambia. *Archives of Neurology*, 2000, 57:414–417.

15. Casanova-Sotolongo P, Casanova-Carrillo P, Rodriguez-Costa J. [A neuroepidemiological study in Beira, Mozambigue]. *Revista de Neurologia*, 2000, 30:1135–1140.

16. Lavados PM et al. [Neurological diagnostics in primary health care in Santiago, Chile]. *Revista de Neurologia*, 2003, 36:518–522.

17. Lester FT. Neurological diseases in Addis Ababa, Ethiopia. *African Journal of Medicine and Medical Sciences*, 1979, 8:7–11.

18. Morrow JI, Patterson VH. The neurological practice of a district general hospital. *Journal of Neurology, Neurosurgery and Psychiatry*, 1987, 50:1397–1401.

19. Kwasa TO. The pattern of neurological disease at Kenyatta National Hospital. *East African Medical Journal*, 1992, 69:236–239.

20. Playford ED, Crawford P, Monro PS. A survey of neurological disability at a district general hospital. *British Journal of Clinical Practice*, 1994, 48:304–306.

21. Lampl C et al. Hospitalization of patients with neurological disorders and estimation of the need of beds and of the related costs in Austria's non-profit hospitals. *European Journal of Neurology*, 2001, 8:701–706.

22. Rose AS. Graduate training in neurology. *Archives of Neurology*, 1971, 24:165–168.

23. *National disease and therapeutic index specialty profile: neurologists*. Ambler, Pa, IMS America Ltd, 1982.

24. Garrison LP: *Physician requirements – 1990: for neurology*. Hyattsville, MD, Office of Graduate Medical Education, US Department of Health and Human Services, 1982.

25. Kurtzke JF. Neuroepidemiology. *Annals of Neurology*, 1984, 16:265–277.

26. Perkin GD. Pattern of neurological outpatient practice: implications for undergraduate and postgraduate training. *Journal of Royal Society of Medicine*, 1986, 79:655–657.

27. Rajput AH, Uitti RJ. Neurological disorders and services in Saskatchewan – a report based on provincial health care records. *Neuroepidemiology*, 1988, 7:145–151.

28. Hopkins A, Menken M, DeFriese G. A record of patient encounters in neurological practice in the United Kingdom. *Journal of Neurology, Neurosurgery and Psychiatry*, 1989, 52:436–438.

29. Perkin GD. An analysis of 7836 successive new outpatient referrals. *Journal of Neurology, Neurosurgery and Psychiatry*, 1989, 52:447–448.

30. Stevens DL. Neurology in Gloucestershire: the clinical workload of an English neurologist. *Journal of Neurology, Neurosurgery and Psychiatry*, 1989, 52:439-46.

31. *UK audit of the care of common neurological disorders*. London, Association of British Neurologists (Services Committee), 1991.

32. Singhal BS, Gursahani RD, Menken M. Practice patterns in neurology in India. *Neuroepidemiology*, 1992, 11:158–162.

33. Boongird P et al. The practice of neurology in Thailand. A different type of medical specialist. *Archives of Neurology*, 1993, 50:311–312.

34. Martin R. [The model of neurological care needs in Valencian community. Commission of the analysis of the quality of SVN]. *Revista de Neurologia*, 1995, 23:1106–1110.

35. Gracia-Naya M, Uson-Martin MM. [Multicentre transverse study of the neurological ambulatory care in the Spanish Health System in Aragon: overall results]. *Revista de Neurologia*, 1997, 25:194–199.

36. Holloway RG et al. US neurologists in the 1990s: trends in practice characteristics. *Neurology*, 1999, 52:1353–1361.

37. Gonzalez Menacho J, Olive Plana JM. [Epidemiology of ambulatory neurological diseases at the Baix Camp]. *Neurologia*, 2001, 16:154–162.

38. Trevisol-Bittencourt PC et al. [The most common conditions in a neurology clinic]. *Arquivos de Neuro-psiquiatria*, 2001, 59:214–218.

39. Herzig R et al. The current availability of neurological inpatient services in post-communist central and eastern European countries. *Neuroepidemiology*, 2003, 22:255–264.

40. Bermejo F et al. [Estimation of the neurological demand in a health-care area of Madrid, Spain (area 11, University Hospital, 12 of October)]. *Neurologia*, 1999, 14:444–451.

41. Carroll C, Zajicek J. Provision of 24-hour acute neurology care by neurologists: manpower requirements in the UK. *Journal of Neurology, Neurosurgery and Psychiatry*, 2004, 75:406–409.

42. Menken M et al. The scope of neurologic practice and care in England, Canada, and the United States. Is there a better way? *Archives of Neurology*, 1989, 46:210–213.

43. Bermejo F. [Demand for neurological services in Spain. Data for a more demanding future]. *Revista de Neurologia*, 1999, 29:673–677.

44. Bartos A et al. Postgraduate Education in Neurology Group at the First European Co-operation Neurology Workshop. Postgraduate education in neurology in Central and Eastern Europe. *European Journal of Neurology*, 2001, 8:551–558.

45. Birbeck GL. A neurologist in Zambia. *Lancet Neurology*, 2002, 1:58–61.

46. Bergen DC. World Federation of Neurology Task Force on Neurological Services. Training and distribution of neurologists worldwide. *Journal of Neurological Sciences*, 2002, 198:3–7.

47. Hooker J et al. Neurology training around the world. *Lancet Neurology*, 2003, 2:572–579.

48. Stevens DL. *Neurology in the United Kingdom: number of clinical neurologists and trainees*. London, Association of British Neurologists, 1996.

49. European Federation of Neurological Societies. *Task force for European subspecialties*. EFNS Newsletter No 3, 2003.

50. Murray CJL, Lopez AD, eds. *Global comparative assessment in the health sector: disease burden, expenditures, and intervention packages* (collected articles from the *Bulletin of the World Health Organization*). Geneva, World Health Organization, 1994.

51. Hauser WA, Hesdorffer DC. *Epilepsy: frequency, causes and consequences*. New York, Demos Press, 1990.

52. Meinardi H et al. on behalf of the ILAE Commission on the Developing World. The treatment gap in epilepsy: the current situation and ways forward. *Epilepsia*, 2001, 42:136–149.

53. Engel J Jr, Pedley TA, eds. *Epilepsy: a comprehensive textbook. Vols. 1, 2 and 3*. Philadelphia, PA, Lippincott-Raven Publishers, 1997: 2976.

54. Reynolds EH, ed. Epilepsy in the world. Launch of the Second Phase of the ILAE/IBE/WHO Global Campaign against Epilepsy. *Epilepsia*, 2002, 43 (Suppl 6):46.

55. Caro JJ, Huybrechts KF, Duchesne I, for the Stroke Economic Analysis Group. Management patterns and costs of acute ischemic stroke: an international study. *Stroke*, 2000, 31:582–590.

56. Feigin VL et al. Stroke epidemiology: a review of population-based studies of incidence, prevalence, and case-fatality in the late 20th century. *Lancet Neurology*, 2003, 2:43–53.

57. Stroke Unit Trialists' Collaboration. Organised inpatient (stroke unit) care for stroke. *Cochrane Database Systematic Review*, 2002, (1):CD000197.

58. Truelsen T, Bonita R, Jamrozik K. Surveillance of stroke: a global perspective. *International Journal of Epidemiology*, 2001, 30 (Suppl. 1):S11–16.

59. Bonita R et al. The global stroke initiative. *Lancet Neurology*, 2004, 3:391–393.

60. Steiner TJ et al. The prevalence and disability burden of adult migraine in England and their relationships to age, gender and ethnicity. *Cephalalgia*, 2003, 23:519–527.

61. Rasmussen BK et al. Epidemiology of headache in a general population – a prevalence study. *Journal of Clinical Epidemiology*, 1991, 44:1147–1157.

62. Scher AI et al. Prevalence of frequent headache in a population sample. *Headache*, 1998, 38: 497–506.

63. *The world health report 2001 – Mental health: new understanding, new hope*. Geneva, World Health Organization, 2001, pp. 22–24.

64. Steiner TJ. Lifting the burden: the global campaign against headache. *Lancet Neurology*, 2004, 3:204–205.

65. Global Parkinson's Disease Survey Steering Committee. Factors impacting on quality of life in Parkinson's disease: results from an international survey. *Movement Disorders*, 2002, 17:60–67.

66. Twelves D, Perkins KSM, Counsell C. Systematic review of incidence studies of Parkinson's disease. *Movement Disorders*, 2003, 8:19–31.

67. Fahn S, Przedborski S. Parkinsonism. In: Rowland LP, ed. *Merritt's textbook of neurology*, 10th edition. Philadelphia, PA, Lipincott Williams & Wilkins, 2000:679–693.

68. Schapira, AHV. Parkinson's disease. *British Medical Journal* 1999, 318:311–314.

69. Prince MJ. The need for research on dementia in developing countries. *Tropical Medicine and Health*, 1997, 2:993–1000.

70. Wimo A et al. The magnitude of dementia occurrence in the world. *Alzheimer's disease and Associated Disorders*, 2004, 17:63–67.

71. The 10/66 Dementia Research Group. Methodological issues in population-based research into dementia in developing countries. A position paper from the 10/66 Dementia Research Group. *International Journal of Geriatric Psychiatry*, 2000, 15:21–30.

72. Bosenquet N, May J, Johnson N. *Alzheimer's disease in the United Kingdom: burden of disease and future care*. London, Imperial College of Science, Technology and Medicine, University of London, 1998 (Health Policy Review Paper 12).

73. The 10/66 Dementia Research Group. Care arrangements for people with dementia in developing countries. *International Journal of Geriatric Psychiatry*, 2004, 19:170–177.

74. Schneider J et al. EUROCARE: a cross-national study of co-resident spouse carers for people with Alzheimer's disease. I: Factors associated with carer burden. *International Journal of Geriatric Psychiatry*, 1999, 14:651–661.

75. Langa KM et al. National estimates of the quantity and cost of informal caregiving for the elderly with dementia. *Journal of General Internal Medicine*, 2001, 16:770–778.

76. Kalache A. Ageing is a Third World problem too. *International Journal of Geriatric Psychiatry*, 1991, 6:617–618.

77. Compston A et al., eds. *McAlpine's multiple sclerosis*, 4th ed. London, Churchill Livingstone, 2004 (in press).

78. Warren S, Warren KG. *Multiple sclerosis*. Geneva, World Health Organization, 2001.

79. Committee on Nervous System Disorders in Developing Countries, Institute of Medicine. *Neurological, psychiatric, and developmental disorders. Meeting the challenge in the developing world*. Washington, DC, National Academy Press, 2001.

LIST OF RESPONDENTS

Country, territory or area	Name	Country, territory or area	Name
Afghanistan	M.S. Azimi	El Salvador	Carlos Antonio Diaz Manzano
Albania	Jera Kruja	Estonia	Janika Kõrv
Algeria	Mahmoud Aït-Kaci-Ahmed Tazir Meriem	Finland	Juha Korpelainen Jorma Palo
Argentina	Roberto Sica	France	Jean-Marc Léger
Armenia	Vahagn Darbinyan	Gambia	Kathryn Burton
Australia	Geoffrey A. Donnan	Georgia	Shota Bibileishvili George Chakhava
Austria	Franz Gerstenbrand	Germany	Michael Strupp
Bahrain	Adel Al-Jishi	Ghana	Paul Ayisu
Bangladesh	Anisul Haque	Greece	Hellenic Neurological Society
Belarus	Victor V. Yevstigneyev	Guatemala	Luis Fernando Salguero
Belgium	M. Van Zandijcke	Honduras	Reyna Durón Marco Tulio Medina Francisco Ramirez
Benin	Dismand Houinato		
Brazil	Marco A. Lana-Peixoto	Hungary	Imre Szirmai
Bulgaria	Irena Velcheva	Iceland	Albert Pall Sigurdsson Sigurlavg Sveinbjörnsdottir
Burkina Faso	Jean Kabore	India	M. Gourie-Devi
Canada	Morris Freedman Donald W. Paty	Indonesia	Jusuf Misbach
Central African Republic	Pascal Mbelesso	Iraq	Sarmed Al-Fahad
China	Wenzhi Wang	Ireland	Michael Hutchinson
China, Hong Kong Special Administrative Region	Richard Kay	Israel	Oded Abransky
Costa Rica	Manuel Carvajal	Italy	Antonio Federico
Croatia	Slava Podobnik Sarkanji Vesna Vargek Solter	Japan	Nobuo Yanagisawa
		Jordan	Ashraf Kurdi
Cyprus	Chris Messis	Kazakhstan	Abenov Bulat
Czech Republic	Zdenek Ambler	Kenya	Renato Ruberti
Denmark	Troels W. Kjær	Lao People's Democratic Republic	Vikham Sengkignavong
Djibouti	Abdoulkarim Said		
Dominican Republic	Juan R. Santoni	Latvia	Ministry of Health Egils Vitols
Ecuador	Fernando Alarcón	Lebanon	Fouad Anton
Egypt	Hassan Hassan ElKalla M. Anwar Etribi	Libyan Arab Jamahiriya	Abduraouf G. Aburkes

Neurology Atlas © 2004 WHO

Country, territory or area	Name
Lithuania	Valmantas Budrys
Luxembourg	Michel Kruger
Madagascar	Marcellin Andriantseheno
Malawi	Gretchen L. Birbeck
Mali	Moussa Traoré
Mexico	Francisco Rubio Donnadieu
Mongolia	D. Baasanjav
Morocco	Mohamed Yahyaoui
Myanmar	Nyan Tun
Netherlands	Marianne de Visser
New Zealand	Andrew Chancellor
Níger	Sadio Barry
Nigeria	M.A. Danesi
Norway	Johan A. Aarli
Oman	Pratap Chand
Pakistan	S.S. Naeem-ul-Hamid
Philippines	Amado M. San Luis
Poland	Urszula Fiszer
Portugal	José Lopes Lima
Puerto Rico	Angel Chinea
Qatar	Ahmad Hamad
Republic of Korea	Seung Min Kim
Republic of Moldova	Vitalie Lisnic
Romania	Ovidio Bajenaru
Russian Federation	Michael Piradov
Saudi Arabia	Saleh M. Al Deeb Fahmi M. Al-Senani
Senegal	Ndiaye Mansour
Serbia and Montenegro	Slobodan Apostolski
Slovakia	Lubomir Lisy
Slovenia	Antón Mesec

Country, territory or area	Name
South Africa	R. Eastman J.A. Temlett
Spain	José Luis Molinuevo Guix Jordi Matias-Guiu
Sri Lanka	J.B. Pieris
Sudan	Daoud Mustafa
Sweden	Sten-Magnus Aquilonius
Switzerland	Julien Bogousslavsky Hans Rudolf Stöckli
Syrian Arab Republic	Ahmad Khalifa
Tajikistan	Sherali Radjabaliev
Thailand	Rawiphan Witoonpanich
Togo	Eric Grunitzky
Tunisia	Najoua Miladi
Turkey	Coskun Ozdemir
Ukraine	Oleksandr E. Kutikov
United Arab Emirates	Jihad Inshasi Gohar Wajid
United Kingdom	Colin Mumford Graham Venables S.J. Wroe
United States of America	Donna C. Bergen Michael F. Finkel Donna M. Honeyman
Uruguay	José Caamaño Alejandro Scramelli
Uzbekistan	Karimov Khamid
Venezuela, Bolivarian Republic of	Rolando Haack
Viet Nam	Le Duc Hinh
West Bank and Gaza Strip	Mazen I. El-Hindi
Yemen	Hesham Awn
Zambia	Gretchen L. Birbeck